EMERGENCY ROOM

LIVES SAVED AND LOST:

Doctors Tell Their
Stories

Edited by **DAN SACHS, M.D.**

 LITTLE, BROWN AND COMPANY *Boston New York Toronto London*

Copyright acknowledgments begin on page 253.

FIRST EDITION

In the interest of protecting patient confidentiality, all of the names, as well as certain identifying characteristics, details of background information, and incidents in these stories have been changed.

Library of Congress Cataloging-in-Publication Data

Emergency room : lives saved and lost: doctors tell their stories / edited by Dan Sachs.
    p.   cm.
    ISBN 0-316-76592-9 (alk. paper)
    1. Emergency physicians — Anecdotes.   2. Emergency medicine — Miscellanea.   3. Hospitals — Emergency services — Miscellanea. I. Sachs, Dan, M.D.
RC87.E535   1996
362.1'8 — dc20   96-8254

10   9   8   7   6   5   4   3   2   1

MV-NY

Published simultaneously in Canada by Little, Brown & Company (Canada) Limited

Printed in the United States of America

FOR *my parents*

CONTENTS

Contents

viii

ACKNOWLEDGMENTS

I am grateful to the physicians who were willing to share their experiences by writing for this collection. I regret that we were unable to publish many of the contributions. I am indebted to the dedicated professionals who taught me my craft, the emergency department staff of Christ Hospital & Medical Center. They run a top-notch residency program! I appreciate the early encouragement of Dr. Raymond Hart, and Little, Brown's Tammy Booth and Mark Chimsky. Catherine Crawford was a wonderful editor. Pamela Marshall's copyediting was right on target. And my agent, Jonathan Matson, did a fine job of hand-holding.

Finally, I am most grateful for the support and tolerance of Joyce Minor.

I enjoy working as a physician in the emergency room, but not for the reason that first drew me to this craft. Initially I was hooked by the stimulation, the adrenaline that quickened my pulse when a critically ill patient demanded intervention. It slapped me awake, like cold water on a drowsy face, made me feel alert, alive. I loved to yell "Clear!" and with paddles shock fibrillating hearts back to life. I yearned to crack a chest, and with rib spreaders expose the heart, burst open by the blunt force of a dashboard. Before sewing split scalp back together, I would rub a gloved finger over the white, bony skull. Since childhood this was my image of doctoring. Saving lives. Blood and guts. Action.

I've sutured and shocked and bloodied myself now thousands of times as an emergency room resident training on the South Side of Chicago. On occasion I am also sprayed by urine, vomit, spit, and other unpleasantnesses. After several years of this work, the adrenaline has lost its potency. My pulse remains steady; I no longer sweat. I do still enjoy the work, though now I am less excited by the heroics of aggressive procedures and cheating death. That has, surprisingly, become almost routine. Instead, I am enthralled by the glimpse this work allows into the lives of patients. It has taken me years to appreciate that my white coat permits me to witness some of the most personal and frightening moments of our existence.

As a medical student, I asked little more from patients than the data needed to complete their charts: chief complaint, past medical history, medications, etc. I was too scared to probe any deeper. For even though I introduced myself as a student, patients took false comfort in the authority of my short white coat. Few realized that the short coat meant novice, so they trusted me as a doctor. The stethoscope looked impressive, but my ears could hardly discern a murmur from a gallop. I was no doctor. Worried they would discover the sham, I did not feel comfortable getting close with patients.

Graduation from medical school placed the awkward initials "M.D." after my name. Into the large pockets of my new, long, white coat, I stuffed the textbooks that would carry me through internship. My neck ached from the tug of these books, but it was an exciting time. Patients would tell me their complaints. I would nod, knowingly, and proceed to the physical exam. This was a comforting ritual, for it suggested that I knew what I was doing. I then would excuse myself from the room to look up their complaints in my medley of texts. Preoccupied with making the right diagnosis to stay credible in the eyes of the supervising attending physician, I paid little attention to anything about my patients beyond their chief complaints.

By year three I grew comfortable managing most of the problems that brought people to the emergency room. I learned to simultaneously juggle back pain, chest pain, headache, and shortness of breath by running through standard algorithms in my head. No longer distracted by the need to look things up or the stress of making the right diagnosis, I finally began to know my patients as more than diagnostic puzzles. I began to view these people as human beings, like myself. I learned to sense their fear, frustration, sadness, annoyance, their exhaustion. The unsuccessful "cardiac arrest in Room Four" became a loving husband and patriarch, whose family I would soon face. The "vaginal bleed in Room Twenty" became a young woman distraught by the notion of losing her baby. I focused less on pathophysiology, more on listening and observing.

For those who take notice amid the hectic bustle of the place, the emergency room displays a rich variety of human drama. Characters of all ages and socioeconomic backgrounds seek relief from problems spanning the range of medical specialties. The course of several hours might bring a father frightened by the chest pain of a heart attack, a teenager screaming in labor, an elderly grandmother rendered speechless by stroke, and a child shot by a stray bullet to his belly. These patients at first feel vulnerable, yet they eventually place their trust in the men and women in white coats. It is a privilege to witness how the courageous struggle with adversity, and the weary surrender to disease. And it is frustrating to confront so many of society's failures all converging on this one place — drug addiction, street violence, child abuse, rape. Physicians try to help. We make some gratifying saves but we also sometimes fail in our attempts to heal.

In an effort to capture for others what it is like to work in the emergency room, I invited doctors with a talent for prose to submit their memorable experiences for this collection. The following vignettes offer a glimpse into the lives of patients and the physicians who care for them. They illustrate what makes the emergency room such a compelling place.

DAN SACHS, M.D.
Senior Resident
Department of Emergency Medicine
Christ Hospital
Chicago

EMERGENCY
ROOM

DUTY

BY *Stewart Massad, M.D.*

For a gynecologist, night call in the ER is always bad — always different, but always bad. And Fridays are the worst.

That Friday night, I began with a girl who carried a gangbanger's jacket and a case of gonorrhea. She studied me with suspicious eyes till I touched her cervix with a culture swab; then she slapped her knees together, hissing a stream of curses that contained all the anger of her thirteen years. I went on to a couple who'd spent two years and God knows how many thousand dollars living out their obsession with pregnancy at the direction of the university's infertility service. I passed all of twenty minutes with them before running her to surgery, showing them on the ultrasound scanner the only baby they'd ever have: just a knot of tissue in a blown-out tube. I saw a party child who asked me to check out her vagina before a weekend of hard use, much as I'd have my mechanic go over my car before a rough trip. A coed from the undergraduate college came in, miscarrying the pregnancy she'd conceived with a guy who'd claimed to have loved her once, though he was nowhere around. She wept the sad and grateful tears of womanhood while I vacuumed out the remnants of misconceptions physical and emotional. I treated a woman with another yeast infection to remind her of the HIV she carried. I saw a fat woman with a discharge, a frightened kid six days late for her period, a case of constipation masquerading as pelvic pain.

Between patients, I fielded the "medical advice" phone calls, which were directed to the ER. "Is it true that douching with pickling salts makes sex better?" the first one asked. "The condom broke: Now what?" "He says I can't get pregnant 'cause it's my first time and my periods haven't started yet." "My boyfriend has these things on his thing. What could they be?"

For variety, I had one obstetric case come through the big pneumatic double doors. The gurney drivers ran her into a cubicle while the nurse shouted "Don't push!" as if repetition and volume could break through the envelope of crack and pain and fear around that thrashing woman. We tore the mother's pants off, cut her panties from her thighs. I pulled the baby from between closed legs. No suction, no stirrups, no drapes, no gown, no pediatrician. I had no prenatal records — if the mother had ever come in to generate any — no idea if the child coming at me was term or premature, normal or not. Nothing was sterile, nothing ready, except the baby. I was all adrenaline as I took the kid by the new-sprouted head, turning the shoulders to fit under the pubic arch, pulling him free as he began to scream, all the while cursing and cursing and cursing to myself.

We all crossed the bar of midnight together: patients, staff, family in the waiting room, the voiceless faces on the lobby TV. Shifting between my two rooms, diagnosing by rote, treating by reflex, I should have been compassionate, but I'd seen too much. I should have evinced empathy, but I'd been up all night in an overheated operating room. I should have radiated confidence and support, but I was too damn tired. There was blood on the cuffs of my slacks and the soles of my shoes. My eyes burned and the skin over my cheekbones felt puffy and dry. My mouth tasted of burnt coffee. I felt as if a stopcock in my heel had been opened and all the optimism and energy had drained out of me. I felt beaten, exhausted, used. All I wanted to do was get through the next case.

That wasn't what I'd gone to medical school looking for, but that had been seven years before. Back then I'd been looking for the sense of satisfaction that follows a job done well. Now all I sensed were desperation and futility. I'd become a doctor for the gratitude I once had seen in the eyes of healed patients. But in the emergency room, the only looks I got were those of anger, denial, resignation, disgust, and annoyance. I'd gone on to residency because I wanted to deliver healthy babies for happy couples. Instead, I'd just held up a husky boy to a mother who lay on a bare black plastic pad with the sheet twisted up under bloody buttocks, who lay with one arm over closed eyes, muttering "Oh, shit" again and again, like it was the mantra for the new age.

When that was done I sat in the back of the charting station and set my head on the countertop. The crowded cacophony around me became nothing more than the hush inside a seashell. Shouts, curses, cries of pain, the shriek of curtain hooks on steel rods, the clank and whine of a self-propelled X-ray machine soothed me like the kitchen sounds of home, where my wife and my daughter were long since sleeping.

A hand on my shoulder pulled me back into the world. I came back from far away and long ago with blue sky and the smell of crushed grass echoing in my head with the taste of a smile.

"Duty," the head nurse reminded me, and when I got up to head back toward my rooms, the only ones with examining tables that hadn't had the stirrups broken off, she said, "No such luck." Retired army, a graduate of the Gulf War, she pointed me firmly toward a cubicle on the ER's trauma side. I glanced at the white message board where all the cases were posted. In the trauma slot was a woman's name and "sexual assault" scrawled out in lazy blue marking ink.

I looked at the nurse, who only shrugged. "The Trauma boys are done with her," she told me. "No fractures, no concussion, nothing deep enough to need sutures. She's all yours." She smiled to see my chagrin, punched me on the shoulder. "Buck up, kid," she said. "Remember: duty." Then she went on.

Duty was a lean, small, determined woman trying hard to sit up straight on the side of a gurney. She was doing well, in spite of the thinness of her shoulders under the worthless hospital gown, in spite of the extra slump life had molded into the curve of her spine, in spite of the air conditioning, in spite of her age. Her gray, wiry hair was done up tightly in a bun, pulled away from her face.

Her face was remarkable. The right side of it was quite normal, an old woman's face, lined, worn, tired so early in the morning and yet determined. But where the right half of her face was a faded brown, the left side was multicolored; and where the features of her right side were sculpted and proud, those on the left were gnomish and broken. There was blood in the white of her eye, and the flesh around the socket was purple, almost black. The skin over her brow was cut, and the new red scab stood out against the mottled tan and blue of her skin. Looking closely, I could make out the marks of fingers on her cheek, just to the side of the split puff of maroon that had been her lips. Her ear was big as cancer, already its violet bruise shot with yellow. She saw me frown and looked at her feet, swinging free in their quiet black oxfords. Then she looked up, bravely trying what must have been a smile, a smile that screwed into a grimace as pain shot through the lumpiness of her face. She looked down at her shoes again.

"Guess I don't look like much," she offered, her response to the dismay she must have seen on my face.

That broke me out of my diffidence: the words of a victim, ashamed of her own disfigurement. I put a hand on her shoulder, took a breath to let the anger leak out of my voice, and shook my head.

"You look fine," I said. I sat down on a steel stool and took the cap off my pen. "What happened?"

She told me. She had told the paramedics, the triage nurse, and then the trauma team, as she would repeat it again to the investigating officer, the prosecutor, the defense attorney, the jury.

It was not a pretty story, though God knows I'd heard it often enough in all its variations. Always it was a woman. Sometimes she was walking where prudence wouldn't have taken her, and sometimes she was at home. Sometimes she was with a man she knew, and sometimes she was alone. Once I'd seen a woman after a gang rape, once after a prom night from hell. I'd seen women from the bad part of town and the best part of the city. I'd seen women raped by drunks, by strangers, by burglars, by husbands. I'd seen women raped with sticks, with knives, with whiskey bottles. I thought I'd seen it all, but this mousy little woman, her calm voice, her twisting hands, her frightened eyes, was almost more than I could stomach.

Still, I was a doctor. I was trained to stomach anything. I sat and wrote down what she told me, prompting when tears welled up and she could not go on. She had been planning to visit her daughter and grandbaby for the weekend, but the child had taken sick, and she'd stayed home. She had gone to bed early, awakened suddenly by the sound of shattered glass spilling across the dining room floor. She had thought at first to hide, but then she'd heard the china crash, heard the hutch overturned, heard him breaking one by one all the souvenir glasses she bought on that one trip to Vegas before her husband had died. She couldn't keep silent. She had yelled. She told him she had a gun. She shouted at him to go. In fact, she did have a gun. A telephone would have helped her more, but that was in the living room. He came up on her from behind while she was rummaging about in the dresser drawer where her husband had kept his pistol.

She'd had only one good look at the man before he was on her. He had hit her with his fist and with the flat of his hand, knocking her against the dresser, bouncing her off the mattress and the footboard. He had asked her for money, told her he'd kill her if she didn't get it. She would have shown him, too, but he kept hitting her, couldn't stop long enough for her to answer him.

For a moment she broke off her story, gingerly dropped the short sleeve of her gown to show me the bruises on her ribs, her shoulder, her arm. He had hit her over and over, she said, calling her bitch, ripping at her nightclothes, tearing at her panties. He was on something. She'd had a boy once — in prison now, and safe. She knew these things. He wouldn't listen when she begged him to stop, didn't stop when he had her down, didn't pause when she screamed at him to think of his own mother.

I wrote it all down. It made for very dry reading. "Patient stated vaginal penetration, attempted anal penetration, no oral penetration. Patient does not recall if ejaculation. Patient denies intercourse since death of husband six years ago. Patient denies knowing assailant, states assailant black, young, short hair with razor part left side, clean-shaven, about 25, about 5'9", no distinguishing marks."

"I bit him, though," she told me. "I bit him good. He put a hand on me to keep me from yelling, and I tried to bite it off." She smiled again at last, remembering. "I tasted blood. He hit me good after that, but he ain't going to forget me — not for a little while yet."

"Will you want to report this to the police?" I asked her.

She looked at me quizzically, as if there were no other course. I explained that if she did or thought she might later, I would have to do a formal examination with evidence collection. I described that for her. I described the police interrogation, the routine ridicule from the defender, the humiliation of trial.

She shrugged and looked past me. "I'm an old woman," she said. "I been through things . . ." Her voice trailed off. She shook her head and fixed me with hard, dark eyes. "Honey, that ain't nothing to what I've seen."

She got down off the gurney unaided. She wrapped a sheet around herself to cover all that remained of modesty as we walked to one of my examining rooms. Though all her clothes might go for evidence, she made the nurse with us bring the clothes piled on a sheet. "You don't know folks around here," she cautioned me. "Take anything ain't nailed down." Once inside she hoisted herself onto the table and put her feet into the stirrups. While I worked, she never spoke, never moved.

I combed through what she had of gray pubic hair and put the gleanings in one envelope, with a few plucked hairs in another, in case the attacker had rubbed off a few of his own. I looked for semen stains on her thighs with a Wood's lamp and found nothing. The skin of her labia was torn along the right side, but the break was clean and superficial, nothing that needed stitches. I took samples of fluid from her vagina for forensic analysis, cultures for venereal diseases, and a drop on a glass slide for myself.

She had no internal lacerations. While I worked, I counseled her about HIV testing. She agreed, wanted everything by the book. There was no need to talk about pregnancy prevention.

I took the glass slide back to the lab. Under the microscope, mixed in with the blood cells, I saw his sperm still swimming.

I felt sick, sick with fatigue and revulsion and hate. I could not go back into her room, where a cop was taking down her story. I stood by the nursing station with my back to a pillar. I wanted a job in the suburbs. I wanted a clean practice, full of virtuous patients who did everything I asked and got better every time I treated them. I wanted to be on a Caribbean beach with the sun in my eyes and the surf lapping at my toes.

To pass the time, I glanced down the list on the patient board: motor vehicle accident, gunshot wound abdomen, multiple stab wounds right chest, left ankle fracture, belly pain, bite wound right hand.

I went cold. For a moment I couldn't catch my breath. Then I caught myself: I had no desire to see my patient's assailant found. It meant nothing to me — or, rather, it meant hours in deposition while some arrogant child from the public defender's office tried to convince a jury that I was incompetent to examine women, more hours at the courthouse while my patients waited and my partners got pissed because I wasn't around to carry my caseload. I reminded myself that I was not involved in this. Identifying the perpetrators of sexual crimes was not my job. My job was to take care of one woman, and perhaps she would be better off without a convicted rapist who knew her name and held a grudge. Anyway, if the guy was such a dope as to come right in to get his hand looked at, the police would find him.

But I knew that wasn't true. I knew the man was almost never found, just like my friends in pediatrics knew the men and women who burned and beat and raped their patients never came to trial. I interrupted my patient's police interview with an order for a shot to treat incipient gonorrhea and fourteen pills out of the samples cabinet for a week's chlamydia treatment. I spoke to the cop and went back outside.

I hoped that the bitten man had been discharged in those few moments, but he had not even been seen yet. He was sitting morosely at the foot of his gurney, looking at the fluorescent lights burn with the steady gaze of a tired addict coming down. His face brightened when I came in.

"About damn time," he said, mistaking me for his doc. He had on no shirt. He was a muscular young man, black, short hair with razor part left side, clean-shaven, about twenty-five, about five foot nine. He had no distinguishing marks, except a welter of scratches and a swollen hand.

I picked up his hand. In the flesh of his palm were multiple punctures, the marks of teeth. When I squeezed, the man jerked his hand away.

"Damn woman," he protested.

"Hurts, doesn't it?" He glared at me. I met his gaze. "How'd it happen?" I asked him.

"Bitch bit me. We was doing it, and she yelling so loud I thought she'd wake the neighbors. Put a hand on her mouth, and she bit me."

I nodded, said nothing. I fingered scratches on his face. "Like it rough, don't you?"

"Women," he scoffed. "They all like it rough." I stepped beside him and ran my hands over scratches on his back. He tried to turn to look at me, but a firm hand kept him facing forward. He obeyed the doctor's touch. Still, he twisted his eyes round and leered. "Bet your bitch like it rough, too, heh? Yeah, like all them white girls."

I felt his neck, as if to examine his trachea and lymph nodes. "What's her name?" I asked. I watched him start to think, watched him begin to worry. "Don't even know her name?" His brows drew together. I smiled for him. "Strange," I lied to him in my softest voice that went suddenly steely, "because she's here tonight, and she knows yours."

I had my fingers at his throat as the panic welled up in his eyes. I had him, but he elbowed me in the ribs. He did not wait to gather up his shirt. He ran straight through the curtains, straight into two men in blue, straight into the cuffs.

I walked past him and through the automatic doors. I sat down on the step the ambulances pull up to, listening to a siren coming in while the pigeons woke. Off east, above the medical center, beyond the church steeples and the telephone poles, the highway ramps and the tenements, morning was a thin line of orange fading into yellow, and I was clean again.

DEBRIDING
THE WOUNDS

BY *Glenn Flores, M.D.*

The infant is crying. He screams. A series of forceful sobs follows until he has no more breath. Just when it seems he has stopped breathing, he takes a long, deep breath and then begins the screaming and sobbing again. He lies on his back, holding his legs in the air, trying to somehow lessen the pain. The entire lower half of his body has been scalded. Flecks of burnt skin and smears of yellow blister fluid stain the pristine whiteness of the paper on the examination table. It is clear that someone has intentionally plunged the boy in scalding hot water.

I look at the boy's emergency room chart. Jamil Johnson is eleven months old. His mother is eighteen years old. The triage nurse has written "bathtub accident" in the Preliminary Diagnosis blank.

Jamil's mother sits in a chair next to the examination table. She is wearing a heavy winter coat. She is tipped back on the chair's rear legs, almost to the point of toppling over. She chews gum slowly, staring at the floor. Her face is turned away from me, but I can see she has a black eye.

I introduce myself.

"Hi," she answers, interrupting the rhythmic chewing.

"How did this happen?" I ask, stroking Jamil's head. He bawls louder.

"I was giving him a bath," she explains, her face expressionless. "I put him in the tub, but then the phone rang. I answered it, and just a few seconds later I heard him crying. When I came back, he had the hot water turned all the way up. So I wrapped him in a towel and called 911."

As she speaks, I turn Jamil gently to inspect his burns. The soft brown skin of his upper body abruptly changes at his waist to raw, oozing redness littered with blisters and seared patches. Only prolonged immersion in scalding hot water could cause these burns. His buttocks and heels were spared by being pressed against cool porcelain; above the characteristic waterline are the splash burns that result when the child struggles to get out of the scalding water.

There is no question that Jamil has been abused. His mother is trying to protect the abuser with her weakly fabricated story. But whom is she protecting?

"Has Jamil had any burns or broken bones before?" I ask, attempting to ascertain how many times he has been abused. He grabs my hand as I speak, unsure whether to pull it toward himself for comfort or push it away in fear.

"Uh-uh," she replies. She bites her lip. "He fell down and hit his head on the coffee table last month, but the doctors said he was okay."

I finish examining Jamil. I take out a strip of tiger stickers that I keep wedged in the last page of my handbook of pediatric drugs, waving it playfully in front of his face. This fails to distract him, and his wailing grows louder with my feeble performance. The suggestion of a child's simple pleasure seems only to intensify his suffering. I paste a tiger sticker on his hand. He glances at the sticker, then at me, and finally at the ceiling, as he continues to cry.

"Jamil's burns are bad, Ms. Robinson," I tell her, bending down on one knee next to her chair. "He's going to have to stay in the

Debriding the Wounds

hospital for a while. We need to make sure that those burns have a chance to heal properly."

She nods, gazing off over her shoulder. I'm not sure if I can see anger, distress, or indifference in the mostly blank look on her face.

"Can I ask you a question?" I say, after getting no further response.

"What?" she says, turning sharply toward me. Her face is only inches away and I feel her throbbing pain. Up close I can see the mashed violaceous skin around her eye socket and the striation of burst capillaries in the white of her eye.

"How did you get the black eye?" I ask her, harboring a few of my own suspicions.

"I got punched," she says, watching Jamil as the nurse takes his temperature.

"Who punched you in the eye?" I ask.

"My boyfriend," she replies, running her fingers over the synthetic fur on her coat collar.

"He's Jamil's father?"

She nods. I notice a three-inch jagged scar on the back of her hand, and next to it a tattoo of the initials "G.K."

"This isn't the first time he's hit you, is it?" I suspect that it's not very difficult for a guy who hits his wife to progress to scalding his kid.

She shakes her head.

"Ms. Robinson," I say, putting my hand on her arm, "this man you call your boyfriend is abusing you. You do not deserve to be beaten. What he is doing to you is also against the law. As a doctor, I'm here to protect you and your child. So the first thing I'm going to do is report him to the police for spouse abuse and have him arrested." I feel my hands involuntarily clenching at my sides.

"Good!" she says, jabbing her index finger in the air. "Throw his sorry ass in jail! I'm tired of taking his crap."

I tuck Jamil's chart under my arm and stand up. "One more

thing, Ms. Robinson," I say, massaging the back of my neck. "Jamil's burns are consistent with someone purposely dunking him in hot water." She turns her head away from me quickly when I say this. "Was this really an accident?"

"Damn, I told you it was!" she snaps, putting her hands on her hips.

"You're not covering for your boyfriend because you're afraid he might do something to you?"

She snaps her head toward me. "Listen!" she says, thrusting an index finger at me. "I told you what happened was an accident. I ain't lyin' to you." She folds her arms and scowls.

"All right, Ms. Robinson, I'm sorry to have to upset you, but it's my duty to make sure we have the facts straight." She brushes at the hem of her coat as I speak.

"I'll be back later to check on Jamil," I tell her. As I walk away, I see her grimace when the intern jabs the needle into Jamil's small, chubby arm.

I sit down in front of the phone at the clerk's desk. Just as I pick up the receiver, I'm startled by a commotion coming from the open automatic doors.

Two security guards are struggling to hold a thrashing drunk in his sixties. His arms flail out like rotors. His legs alternately collapse, then kick violently. "I'm going to kill all of you SOBs! *All* of you!" he screams.

Another security guard walks quickly through the automatic doors. "You're covering kids, right?" he says to me through the open window in front of the desk. He breathes heavily from exertion.

"Yes," I answer, rising from my seat and replacing the telephone receiver.

"We need your help. We got one very angry father out here who wants to know what's happening to his son."

Jamil's father is about six foot two and 250 pounds. He has three hoop earrings in each ear and a small diamond stud in his nose. He wears a black sweat suit with blue stripes. Two beepers are clipped to his waistband. Three thick gold chains are draped around his neck. They clink with his abrupt movements. Two equally large security guards stand on either side of him, eyeing him from a respectful distance.

I reach out my hand. "Hi. I'm — "

"Are you the doctor?" he shouts, thrusting his head toward me.

"Yes, sir. I'm Dr. Flores, the pediatrician." I can't say that I've actually been afraid of many people that I've met, but this man is one of them. People with no limits scare me, people who can express themselves only through violence. I sense that in him.

I extend my hand. He gives it a perfunctory shake. "How's my boy? Is he all right?" He holds his hands in half fists at his sides.

"He's got some pretty bad burns," I explain, sighing. "He's going to have to stay in the hospital for a while."

"Aw, man!" he says, burying his face in his hands. He begins breathing heavily through his teeth. "I'm gonna *get* that bitch," he hisses in a low, harsh voice. He pulls his hands slowly down his face, then clenches them into fists which he presses against his chest. "How could she do this to him? I'm gonna kick her ass!"

"Mr. Johnson — " I say.

"Where's my son?" he interrupts. "I gotta see him right now. Where *is* he?" He glares at me. A droplet of spittle is perched on his lower lip.

"Relax, Mr. Johnson. He's safe," I tell him calmly. "The burn doctor is on his way over to take care of the wounds." He becomes slightly calmer when he hears this. He stares at the floor.

"Your wife says you punched her in the eye," one of the guards says, stepping toward him, his hand clutching his nightstick. "Is that correct?"

Jamil's father stares at the floor for a few seconds, saying nothing. I see his nostrils flare just before he lunges at the guard, throwing him hard against the wall. The other guard steps back quickly, pulling out his walkie-talkie to call for backup. Jamil's father bursts down the hall toward the main hospital. I hear his chains swishing and clinking.

What a fool that security guard is! I was hoping to gain the father's trust to obtain some vital information about what happened to Jamil and his mother. I glower at the guard as he speaks into his walkie-talkie. He glances at me, then stares at the floor, scratching his neck. He puts his walkie-talkie away, looks at his partner, and the two of them go lumbering after Jamil's father.

I return to check on Jamil. A burn resident is debriding his wounds, cutting the dead skin away from the live. I remember learning to debride as a medical student, gently removing foreign material and dead tissue until surrounding healthy tissue is exposed. Jamil screams, thrashing his head; one hand clutches the resident's sleeve. Burn patients say this process inflicts the most excruciating pain they have ever experienced. I look at the small pile of dead skin accumulating on the stainless steel tray that holds an array of scalpels, forceps, and probes. Watching the damaged skin being ripped away from the viable, it strikes me that often the worst part of being hurt physically or emotionally is not the initial injury, but the process of treating it.

"I just spoke to Jamil's father," I tell Ms. Robinson, who stands with her back to Jamil, staring at the floor, her hands buried in her pockets.

"Oh, no!" she shouts, wheeling around. "Does he know about Jamil?"

"Yeah," I reply, watching her pace back and forth, scratching her left forearm furiously.

Something is not right here. What kind of question is that? Of course he knows about Jamil, since he burned the kid, didn't he?

Debriding the Wounds

"Why?" I ask her. "Is something wrong?"

"He ain't coming in here, is he? *Please* don't let him in here." She is crying. "He's gonna kill me when he sees Jamil."

"Right now he's loose in the hospital, but he doesn't know where the two of you are, and the security guards are going to take him into custody." I put my hand on her back. "Don't worry. I promise we won't allow anything to happen to you or Jamil. The nurses will move both of you to a secluded room." I look up at the nurse who is assisting the burn resident. She nods, putting down a roll of gauze, and leaves to make the arrangements. "Right now I'm going to call the police to have him arrested."

As I walk toward the telephone, I notice the security guard Jamil's father had pushed. He is standing in the corner, speaking into his walkie-talkie.

"Have you taken him into custody?" I ask him.

"Not yet. The suspect was last seen heading toward the burn unit." He glances at me quickly, blushing, trying to hide behind a barrage of police jargon. "Several security guards are in pursuit and should be apprehending him shortly."

"I expect him to be arrested and charged with assaulting his wife," I say to him sternly.

"We won't be able to do that, sir," he says, then speaks into his walkie-talkie.

I telephone the local police right away. No one has notified them.

I complete the paperwork for Jamil's admission to the hospital. I describe meticulously the dimensions, degree, and location of each burn, knowing that Child Welfare and the courts all view this as a key legal document. I look at the standard hospital burn sheet, contemplating the outlines of a supine and prone child provided to illustrate the burns. Below the child's outlines are adult outlines. I wonder what Jamil will be like when he is older. Whom will he blame for his scars: his mother? his father? the building superintendent? chance? himself?

GLENN FLORES, M.D.

One of the security guards taps me on the shoulder. "Dr. Flores?"

"Yes," I say, closing Jamil's chart.

"The police have Jamil Johnson's father in handcuffs at the emergency room entrance and would like to have a word with you."

I see a policeman standing at the door, waiting to escort me.

"This gentleman has a number of priors," the policeman tells me as we walk toward the entrance. "It looks like he's a crack dealer. He just got out on bail two weeks ago."

The automatic doors to the foyer open and I see Jamil's father. He is sitting on the floor, his hands cuffed behind him. Three police officers are standing around him in a semicircle. One is filling out a report.

"Doc," he says as soon as he notices me. "How's my boy?"

"He's doing better. We cleaned up all the burnt skin and we gave him medicine for the pain," I explain, crouching down in front of him.

"Is he gonna have bad scars?" he asks, staring out the glass doors at the flashing blue lights of the police cars.

"It's difficult to say at this point. We have to see how his burns heal."

"*She* did this to Jamil," he says, shaking his head.

"What do you mean?" I ask, a little surprised. I figure this is his twisted logic, that she "made" him do it.

"She burned him in that hot water on purpose. She got this messed-up idea that I was running around with all these other women. She didn't like that I was out all the time. You know, a guy's gotta make money. I'm not proud of what I do, selling drugs, but there ain't much else I can do," he says, sniffling twice loudly. "But I always treated her right. I gave her money. I took care of Jamil. He's my son, and I love him," he says, looking at the ceiling for a moment.

A gust of cold air chills me as the outside doors open. A few

Debriding the Wounds

people file in on their way to the waiting room, staring at him as they slowly walk by.

"Last night I came by and we had this really bad fight. She said, 'Don't you leave this apartment!' I said, 'Why not? I got work to do.' She said, 'You walk out that door and you gonna regret it. I'm gonna do somethin' bad — real bad — to Jamil. So you better not be goin' nowhere!' " He scratches his chin with his shoulder. "Man, that really ticked me off. So I popped her one in the eye. I told her, 'Don't you ever lay a hand on my boy, or I'll kill you!' I know I shouldn't have popped her in the face, but I was real mad when she said she was gonna do somethin' to my boy. I told her, 'When I come back, I'm taking Jamil away to my mother's.' She said, 'Oh no, you're not! Don't you dare, or you'll be sorry! I'll hurt Jamil *real* bad.' "

"So you're saying that Jamil's mother scalded Jamil on purpose?" I ask, still skeptical.

"I *know* she did. She called me just before she came to the hospital and said, 'I told you not to leave me! This is your fault! Look what you made me do to him!' "

"Has she ever done anything like this before?" I ask, wondering whether he might be telling the truth.

"Look, she's just a horrible mother. That apartment is disgusting. I get tired of that mess. She never changes Jamil's diaper, and she goes out partying all the time, leaving him alone and everything. Half the time I come over and change the kid's smelly diaper that's been on for at least a day or two. My mother even called Child Welfare on her once, but they didn't do nothin', just asked some questions."

I'm in shock. The mother's story and attitude bothered me, and what the father says is making sense.

"We'll definitely look into what you've told us," I tell him.

"Please, Doc, he's my only son."

He starts squirming, trying to free his hands. Two policemen hold him down.

"Hey, why they got me cuffed like this? Why'd they arrest me?"

"You hit your wife," I tell him. "It's against the law, even if she did what you said."

He glowers at me, breathing heavily through his teeth. "It's your fault! All this is your fault! I blame you! I'm gonna get you!"

I step back, stunned by his outburst. The policeman who had escorted me says, "We'll call you later to ask you some questions," then runs outside to help.

I walk back to the emergency room. I peer through the small window of the examination room door. Jamil is still screaming. A nurse strokes his hair, trying to soothe him. His mother sits in a chair, staring out a window at passing cars, her back to her child. She looks bored.

I open the door. Jamil looks up at me but continues to cry.

"Shhh, little guy," I say to him, taking his small hand in mine and giving it a little squeeze. "Everything is going to be all right."

I turn to speak to his mother. She is still gazing out the window.

"They've taken your boyfriend into custody," I tell her.

"They got him?" she says, and as she turns to look at me I see a tight-lipped smile form on her lips. "They put him in jail?"

"Yes. But before they took him away, he told me everything that happened," I say to her. I can feel my eyes squinting in disgust. "You did this to your son, didn't you?"

She drops her head and stares at the floor. She glances at Jamil for just a moment, then stares at the floor again and slowly nods her head.

"ARE YOU SATISFIED, THOMAS BECKET?"

BY *David Feldshuh, M.D.*

My patient was *dead*. He had no pulse. He wasn't breathing. His pupils were wide and staring. As I sat listening to the paramedic's radio report, I was relieved. I now knew exactly what I had to do. I had to bring him back to life.

An hour before, he had walked into a deserted auto repair shop. The garage manager hadn't called him until late Saturday afternoon, pleading that they needed all their lifts for the Monday rush. Even at time and a half he had other things to do. Today was the day he had set aside to repair the cedar railing he had built around the family's new outdoor patio.

The service area was cool, quiet, and empty. High windows projected the morning sun into a sequence of light-dark-light-dark across the width of the work area. He stood for a moment counting the hydraulic lifts. Six. All at ground level except for the second lift at the far end of the rectangular garage. This lift was caught in midair and slightly tilted in his direction like an airplane turning in final approach. Perched on it was a tan Mercedes. They hadn't told him that the lift had broken with a car still on it.

He turned the chrome deadbolt on the glass service door, not expecting to be disturbed by customers on a Sunday morning but wanting to make sure that no one wandered in thinking the repair shop open.

He moved down the line closer to the broken lift. The Mercedes 450 SL floated six feet above the painted gray garage floor. The car listed toward him about ten degrees.

The broken hydraulic lift was slightly larger than the others and was intended for the heavier foreign cars. It was an older model with two columns. The central lifting column was shiny and slick with oil. Next to it stood a smaller, rusted auxiliary column about three inches in diameter. Both columns disappeared into the floor below. The rusted column had an indentation at its base from which a safety catch could be extended to the floor. This safety leg would stop the lift from descending more than a few inches if the compressed air failed to hold it. He quickly noted that this mechanism was missing. In its place someone had drilled a half-inch hole through the auxiliary column at a height of about three feet. Inserted into this hole was a thin, rusted metal rod about fifteen inches long. He shook his head in disbelief. The height of the rod was a mistake. The lift could descend a full three feet prior to being stopped by the metal rod as it contacted the garage floor.

He arranged his tools in a fan pattern on the floor. He liked to work when it was quiet, an infrequent luxury. The garage was a pleasant place, he thought. Ordered and clean.

Freeing the cover plate at the top of the lift's central column he examined the mechanism, searching for a gasket leak that might account for the unexpected stutters that the garage manager had reported. He replaced the most worn gasket and tested the mechanism. The jack groaned, shuddered, and then began to ascend in fits and starts, moving unpredictably and with visible effort. Clearly he had not found the problem and would have to check the compressed air lines in the pit below. Moving underneath the car, he glanced at the metal safety rod in the auxiliary column.

Twenty-five minutes later, after replacing two hose connectors, he emerged from under the car and moved to the brass control lever at the side of the stall in order to test the lift. As he pushed the lever down, the lift began to shake and to his surprise eased into a controlled descent. As he pushed the lever down again to increase the compression and force the lift to rise, he heard an unexpected whine. He was momentarily afraid that the lift would crash to the floor but quickly reasoned that even the inadequate, homemade safety rod had enough strength to arrest its slow descent.

Instinctively, he pulled back two steps keeping his right hand on the control lever. The stuttering descent accelerated as the Mercedes wobbled on the lift tracks. The large central and thin auxiliary columns began to disappear much too rapidly into the floor below. There goes my Sunday, he thought, visualizing the Mercedes bouncing off the lift tracks from a height of three feet and crash-landing on the garage floor.

This could have happened except that the metal rod in the auxiliary column was slightly bent where it protruded. It was rusted and brittle and this stress point was exactly where it contacted the metal sleeve in the floor that surrounded the auxiliary column as it disappeared. The sleeve cut through the safety rod, flipping it violently and launching it into an arrowlike flight across the garage floor in the direction of the control lever.

A few inches lower and he would have suffocated with a ruptured trachea. A few inches to the left and it would have been a close call, to be talked about and recalled perhaps with a wry smile or a whistle of relief. But the velocity of the steel rod was fast enough that it didn't deviate from its precise trajectory. The metal rod raced unflinchingly toward him.

His eyes saw it before his body could recoil in self-protection. The metal rod pierced the muscle layers of his neck and embedded in the spinal bones with a muffled thud.

His first sensation was a tug at the right side of his neck. It hurt, but the end of the rod was sharp. The rod had somersaulted in the air and the pinched, compressed end had made a clean entrance wound just below his chin. He felt some pain but mostly surprise, and it wasn't pain that told him that something was very wrong. Looking down obliquely past his nose he could see the protruding metal. The incongruous visual sensation of the rusted rod fixed horizontally and pointing past his right shoulder frightened him. The metal rod obediently responded to each small move of his neck, catching his eye whenever he turned his head.

As he ran to the service door, he raised his right hand to still the quivering metal arrow. He had to let go of the rod to unlock the door. That's when he saw the blood on the chrome deadbolt. His hand was slippery with blood and he had to struggle with both hands to turn the lock. To his surprise, he needed both arms to pull the door open. Once outside, he could no longer run.

Searching the empty street for help, he saw a Walgreens sign and headed for it. Three more steps, he said, pushing himself to stay calm and in control. He counted his steps. "One, step; two, step; three, step." He could feel his shirt sticking to him.

The heat rising off the hot, black pavement told the circulatory channels of his legs and arms to steal precious blood from an already starving heart and brain. "One, step; two, step; three, step." By the time he cleared the perimeter of the garage parking lot, his shirt was dyed red and the world had begun to spin in a fog of sight and sound. He willed his legs to walk. "One, step . . . two, step . . ."

Soon he would begin to die from the top down: first thought and speech; then sight and sound; then breathing; until finally, deprived of oxygen, the heart would flutter, stumble, and still.

But the heart is a shrewd operator: It pumps blood into the body's largest artery, the aorta, only to reclaim immediately some of this blood through smaller channels backtracking from the aorta to the heart itself.

"Are You Satisfied, Thomas Becket?"

The brain watches out for itself as well. When threatened it commands the body to bow low so that the heart won't have to pump straight up against gravity. It was this royal command that caused his body to stagger and fall to the ground.

He was crawling now, thinking one-word thoughts: "arm, lift, window, jack, wet, hot, blood, eyes." As the brain's higher functions failed, thought disconnected. The Walgreens sign splintered into flying *W*'s and *e*'s. Bright halos infused his visual field. As his hearing shut down, the chugging sound of a diesel truck struggling up a nearby hill receded into a tunnel of silence. He tried to shout.

The Walgreens window diagonally across the street from the garage catered to the older population that lived in three nearby nursing homes. Walkers, toilets on wheels, crutches, and canes created a metal maze of competing geometric shapes through which the pharmacist saw a faltering figure. He first thought the man was drunk. But it was a Sunday morning and he wondered at the glint of metal that reflected the already blistering sun. Trying to fit the fleeting image into a configuration that would seem familiar, the pharmacist recalled thinking, A drunk with a rusty, metal necklace. But he knew that drunks stagger. This figure was tight and desperate to stand as if he were using all his energy to lock his faltering knees. Later the pharmacist remembered thinking that the man's jittery movements looked like a flickering lightbulb. As the pharmacist came out onto the sidewalk, he saw the figure become very still for a few moments, fall to his hands and knees, and gently lie down as if to rest on a blanket of his own blood. Running toward the injured figure, he heard a weak shout: "Ice."

The ambulance arrived within three minutes to find a heart still beating but rapidly and without enough force to compensate for the significant amount of blood loss. The skin was cool and wet. Blood pressure, measuring the heart's efficiency and power, was falling. The supine figure, now a new patient, moaned, "All ice," as he moved in and out of consciousness. I learned later that afternoon that his wife's name was Alicia.

If the patient couldn't scream in terror for his own life, the ambulance could: *da-DAH, da-DAH, da-DAH,* a two-octave decibel war with itself. I don't remember what I was doing when I received the radio call: a sore throat? a low back pain? one of those minor inconveniences that result from having a body in inevitable competition with other organisms, human and nonhuman alike.

Da-DAH, da-DAH, da-DAH, blared the speaker as I sat down to take the call and the ambulance identified itself. My mind began to race: Whatever happened to the old-time siren, the smooth, wailing siren, the kind that sounded sequentially, plaintive and polite, one sound respectfully fading before the next introduced itself? *RAHHHHhhhhhhhhhhhh . . . RAHHHHhhhhhhhhhhhh . . .* No. Now it's *da-DAH, da-DAH, da-DAH.*

Wake up, I demanded. Concentrate. Focus. Listen. Take a breath and listen. In a calm radio voice I responded, "Ten-four, I copy. Go ahead, twenty-eight."

The paramedic report floated over the static: "We've got a thirtyish, white male found in a pool of blood with a metal rod sticking from his neck; no witnesses to the injury; initial blood pressure 95, pulse 140; patient is confused." As the paramedics continued, I noted that the patient's blood pressure was falling in spite of two large IVs pouring fluid into his depleted circulatory system.

What's going on here? I wondered. Was this guy speared? In the neck? Was it a spear attack?! In front of a Walgreens?

Concentrate. I started asking questions: "Any other injuries? Is his neck immobilized? How much blood loss? Did the metal rod penetrate the skull? Was he shot also?"

At this point a tenuous situation turned worse as cells, tissues, organs all became ravenous for oxygen and began thirsting for blood. With little to supply, the heart accelerated, pumping precious dregs as fast as it could squeeze itself empty, refill, and squeeze again. But the heart was pumping so fast that it had no time to allow blood to fill its chambers before the next beat. Less and less blood was ejected into the system and, finally, the heart began to starve itself.

Deprived of blood, the sinus node located in the heart's upper chamber and responsible for sparking the heart to beat began to flicker and fade. In response, chemical messengers, molecular Paul Reveres, raced along the heart's rough muscular surface and sounded the alarm: "The heart's main power source is failing. The spark of life is weakening." Scattered throughout the heart muscle are other self-starting sparks, placed there by nature for just such an emergency. They wait like fireflies ready to ignite, ready to serve.

And they did. All at once independent life sparks desperately tried to jump-start the dying motor of the body. From every part of the heart's geography, minute electrical explosions erupted commanding local pockets of muscle to contract. "Pump blood. Now," they screamed. Small sections of heart muscle contracted in response but without sympathy or coordination. In anarchy, the heart began to quiver like jittery Jell-O. The cardiac monitor etched a chaotic line, a squiggling worm in seizure. This twisted, disordered line well represented the heart's large chambers, the ventricles, as they uselessly fibrillated. The heart, though still alive, had effectively shut down.

Da-DAH, da-DAH, da-DAH. The siren was endless and the paramedic's report brief: "He's in ventricular fibrillation."

"Defibrillate, two hundred watt-seconds," I respond, automatically.

"Two hundred watt-seconds," they repeat. "Ten-four." They have received the order, are confirming and will follow it.

I wait. Not for long.

"No change. Still V-fib."

DAVID FELDSHUH, M.D.

"Defibrillate three hundred, then three-sixty watt-seconds."

"Three hundred then three-sixty, ten-four," they acknowledge.

I wait, grateful for small favors. At least his heart still has some electrical life in it even if it is only squiggling uselessly. At least his heart hasn't completely stopped. At least he's not in asystole.

"Asystole," the paramedics report right on cue. "We've begun CPR."

"Where are you?" I ask.

"At the door. We'll be in in thirty seconds."

"Ten-four," I acknowledge.

I swivel my chair from the radio and look into the inquiring eyes of the charge nurse.

"How dead is this patient?" they seem to ask me.

"Semidead," I respond silently.

Even with CPR in progress, I have little time before irreversible brain damage will transform my patient into a body without a soul. His personness — his feelings, insights, ambitions, opinions — the constellation of traits that make him unique, already hovers tentatively, a fragile mist in the crevices of a stunned brain. Without oxygen and sugar even this mist will soon evaporate, leaving eyes that might open, but only into vacancy.

As my own pulse begins to rise, I know I have only one ally: the undeniable reality that my patient's body is shutting down forever. This fact alone demands action so definite that all shadows of doubt have to be banished. Something drastic has to be done and with total confidence.

"Follow the yellow brick road." The *Wizard of Oz* theme song starts to dance in my head. Whenever I find myself at this point in a case, ready to choose a course of action, that song plays with me. "Follow the yellow brick road. Follow the yellow brick road." It was a squeaky, singsongy voice.

Quiet. Breathe, I command myself. "What's the diagnosis?" I whisper. The cross-examination has begun. Myself against myself.

"Are You Satisfied, Thomas Becket?"

29

Only a zebra hunter would guess that this case was anything other than what it obviously was: a healthy man with a rod sticking out of his neck who has lost so much blood that his heart has stopped. (If you were in horse country and you heard the pounding of hooves, you might guess that horses would be coming over the hill. In medicine, most would agree with you. Others would conclude, unlikely as it might be, that a herd of zebras would soon appear. Zebra hunters propose the most obscure diagnosis for the most obvious of cases. Unfortunately, they are sometimes right.)

I try out my diagnosis on the nurse: "Traumatic arrest."

She nods her head.

"I'm sure his heart's healthy," I continue. "He's just lost so much blood that there's nothing left to pump."

She waits for more. She's listening!

I build my case: "And his heart stopped less than a minute ago. And before that he had a blood pressure."

"The paramedics are wheeling him in now, Doctor," the secretary calls from the reception room.

But how aggressive was I willing to be? He was dead and I could leave him dead.

Did I really want to cut into his chest and then have to answer all those questions: "What were you thinking about anyway? What did you think you could do? Why did you spend all that money on a dead man?" And did I really want to wrestle with the angel and probably lose?

But if I won? I could win. I was two weeks from finishing my residency and at top form. This was one I could win.

"Thoracotomy tray, please." I tried to sound relaxed, even casual, as in, "Pass the salt, please." "Follow the yellow brick road," the song chirped in my head. I squelched it with a muffled cough. "I'm going to open his chest, perform internal cardiac massage, compress the aorta, and divert whatever blood remains to the heart and head. In the meantime let's pour fluid into him. Let's get that heart beating."

"Okay." The nurse sounds cheery. Almost singsongy. "Follow the yellow brick road." That kind of voice.

"I'm going to crack his chest," I repeat with a bit more volume just to make sure that I can no longer retreat. "I'll intubate, seven-point-five tube. Call Respiratory Therapy. Six units type and cross-match. Call Neurosurgery. Call Vascular Surgery. Convert that eighteen-gauge to an eight French. Fluid wide open. Begin O-negative blood as soon as it arrives. Let's stabilize that rod." The orders come easily. I'm pumped.

The patient is lying on his back. I huddle over his face, open his mouth, and with the bright light of a laryngoscope begin to search the dark recesses behind his tongue for landmarks to guide me in placing the breathing tube. For a moment I feel as if I'm alone in a small secluded cave. Finally, the vocal cords come into view and I gently advance the tip of the tube through them and into the trachea. As I bend over to check the lungs for breath sounds to assure me that the tube is correctly placed, I feel a new presence at my back.

"Dr. Terence?" I ask over my shoulder.

"Present," he replies amiably, a hovering cherub, speaking the lines of a schoolboy. Dr. Terence is a man in his fifties, an immensely experienced chest surgeon, congenial, large, with an extremely precise frontal hair transplant. I have heard of him and spoke to him once when I was caring for a patient with a collapsed lung. ("Less than ten percent; no problem," he told me optimistically in his "ain't the world great?" lilt.)

My mouth shifts into overdrive: "Thirty-two-year-old, white male." (Why did I say that? He can see it's a male, and that he's white; slow down.) "He had vital signs in the ambulance; he arrested less than one minute before he arrived."

"Uh-huh," Dr. Terence offers helpfully.

For the first time, I notice that Dr. Terence is wearing tennis shorts. And a white shirt with an alligator.

"Traumatic arrest," I continue anxiously. "I was preparing to do a thoracotomy." Though I'm only two weeks from finishing my residency, the habit of deferral and approval-seeking is strong. I am a doctor, yes. I just don't quite feel like one.

"Thoracotomy," Dr. Terence says, smiling. "Uh-huh," he adds.

I now notice the new white tennis shoes that Dr. Terence is wearing. Using precise deductive processes, I conclude that prior to his arrival, Dr. Terence had been playing tennis.

"Here's the thoracotomy tray," I add nonsensically. As if he didn't know what a thoracotomy tray was. Or was blind.

Dr. Terence continues to, well . . . watch.

I pick up the scalpel as if to prove my point. Thoracotomy. I'm going to do a thoracotomy. Get it?

What's he waiting for?

"Two minutes," the nurse announces. CPR has been in progress for two minutes, and is continuing. This provides temporary and partial circulation at best.

"Two minutes," I mumble.

I steal a glance at Dr. Terence, searching for the smallest suggestion of intent: a subtle move, a minute gesture, anything that would confirm that Dr. Terence, a chest surgeon after all, was going to become captain of this rapidly sinking ship. He shifts his considerable weight from left leg to right leg but holds his ground.

I inhale sharply and see Dr. Terence as if for the first time. My heart rate is about 120. Dr. Terence lopes along at something closer to 70. I'm sweating through the arctic air conditioning in the ER. Dr. Terence is cool and dry: relaxed, arms crossed, sporty, and most of all, content.

Eeeeyoouuuuuuu, I scream, silently. Well, too short for a scream.

More like a yelp. I realize that Dr. Terence is waiting for me. *He's* waiting for *me*. And he's going to *watch*.

Airway, breathing, circulation, I jam silently to myself. The lord is my shepherd. Anything. Something. Onto the roller coaster. Here I go. Breathe. Concentrate. Focus. Repeat. Ribs. Count. Find the nipple. That's the rib I'm looking for. The nipple I can find. I can find a nipple. Calm down. Breathe. That's the nipple, right? He's dead, isn't he? Pupils fixed and dilated? I check. Yes.

"Two minutes, fifteen seconds," the nurse adds helpfully.

Do it, I exhort my weaker part. Resurrect him. Cut into his thorax, search for his heart and squeeze it. You've performed a dozen thoracotomies.

But none of those patients lived. The lord-high cross-examiner has reappeared.

And I know that my decision might injure everything below the level of my patient's heart. Compressing the aorta presents that risk. Blood will be shunted away from the kidneys and lower extremities to supply the heart and brain. The kidneys will be deprived of desperately needed oxygen. I glance at the metal rod protruding from the patient's neck and then at the metal rod I will use to press the aorta firmly but gently against the bones of the spinal column. The rod of devastation and the rod of salvation look surprisingly similar.

I look down. His ribs form a pale cage around his heart. Just below the level of the nipple I feel for the fifth rib. A rack of roast beef momentarily dances in my head. With my index finger I trace the course of the fifth rib from breastbone to backbone. I will have to cut below this line in order to open the chest like a divine book.

"Stop compressions," I order. The nurse moves away from the chest as I quickly clean and drape the area closest to the incision point.

I pick up the scalpel. Holding it in my right hand between

"Are You Satisfied, Thomas Becket?"

thumb and index finger, I examine the blade attached to it. Its cutting edge curves gently, a blade intended to slice with smooth, long strokes.

I rehearse the move once, then again, and again: a downward, curving stroke to follow the rib from just below the nipple to where the patient's back meets the bloodied white sheet on the stretcher. I have to stay close to the top of the sixth rib so as not to cut the arteries and nerves located under the fifth rib less than an inch above.

I return to my catechism: ABC — Airway, Breathing, Circulation — and check each off in my mind. The patient is intubated. Breath sounds can be heard from both lungs. Fluid is pouring in through two intravenous lines to restore the patient's circulation. O-negative blood, blood that can be given to any recipient, is on the way. There is nothing more to do except what needs to be done.

"Two minutes, thirty seconds," the nurse reports. Or has it been a year?

Dr. Terence makes a move. Backward. Out of range of any accidental spatters of blood.

I will my hand to touch scalpel blade to skin. I command myself: Cut. Now. Cut.

The fresh blade is sharp and moves elegantly along the gentle curve of the rib like a skier gliding down a frozen mountain pass. The skin opens and gapes slightly, inviting a deeper cut. I return to my starting point and place the blade. I know I have to use more pressure on this stroke to get through the muscle layers. I press firmly following the red line of my first incision.

Once more. Careful with this one. You don't want to push the blade into the lung, I say to myself. I slide the blade one last time along the slope of the ribs, and the muscles pull apart like an accordion opening. I can see the tip of the left lung rising and falling with the breaths breathed into it by the respiratory therapist.

DAVID FELDSHUH, M.D.

"Spreader, please." I place the spreader like a reverse vise between the fourth and fifth ribs. Turn, push, turn, push . . . there. The ribs open enough to put a hand through.

"Three minutes, thirty seconds," the nurse announces.

Reaching into an open chest is like entering a holy place. My hands disappear below the shadow cast by the chest wall. I feel a momentary sense of relief when my hands encircle the heart: right hand underneath, left hand on top. What would have happened if I couldn't find it? The heart patiently rests in my right hand. Totally still. Quiet. I start to squeeze the silent heart, compressing it between my palms. Squeeze-release, squeeze-release.

At this point, I introduce myself to Dr. Terence. Perhaps I think he might offer some confirmation of my technique. Or at least some thoughts about something. Or perhaps I'm just in need of companionship.

"By the way, I'm — "

"Oh, I know who you are."

"You do?" Squeeze-release, squeeze-release.

Dr. Terence perks up. He seems to grow decidedly animated.

"Oh, yes, I know who you are. Very much so."

He knows me. I'm surprised but pleased.

"Your reputation precedes you," he adds cryptically.

Now, that comment cut two ways. I couldn't remember if I had been on rounds with Dr. Terence and done well or taken care of one of his patients and performed poorly. There were two instances in my brief medical career when experienced doctors heard of a small positive contribution I had made to one of their patients. I hoped that this was instance number three.

I continue carefully to compress the heart resting in my hands. It remains lifeless.

" 'Are you satisfied, Thomas Becket?' " Dr. Terence suddenly quotes in a strange, oval voice.

"Are You Satisfied, Thomas Becket?"

I turn briefly toward him. Was he talking to me?

He says it again in even rounder tones: " 'Are you satisfied, Thomas Becket?' *Becket*. You directed *Becket*," Dr. Terence adds by way of explanation. "I've enjoyed a number of the plays you've directed here in town," he continues. "I remember reading that you had decided to go to medical school. Why in the world would you want to do that?"

Why indeed? I wonder.

I had, it was true, acquired a local reputation as a professional theater director prior to going to medical school, and I had directed the play *Becket* by French playwright Jean Anouilh. This wasn't, however, an achievement I had been mulling over at that particular moment.

"The first scene," Dr. Terence continues smoothly. "I loved the first scene." Squeeze-release, squeeze-release.

"Uh-huh," I answer. Two could play the "uh-huh" game.

" 'Are you satisfied, Thomas Becket?' The first line of the play. Am I right?" He was clearly delighted with his recollection.

"Right," I mumble. Squeeze-release, squeeze-release. Nothing. The heart is doing nothing. I check the position of the rod on the compressed aorta. I reposition it slightly. A nurse holds the rod in place as I move my hands back to the patient's heart. I can feel against my hands the left lung inflating and deflating guided by the steady rhythm of the respiratory therapist. I'm starting to sweat at the top of my ears. That's where I always start to sweat when panic begins to enshroud me.

"Pride before the fall, eh?" Dr. Terence concludes grandly.

"What?" I'm startled and suddenly on guard.

"Becket's pride. Too proud. Pride before God." Dr. Terence was certainly having a wonderful conversation. "Am I right?"

"Sure, right." I'm relieved. For a moment I had thought he was talking about me.

Squeeze-release. Squeeze-release. My hands continue to work and hope.

"Good job," Dr. Terence says, bobbing his head in affirmation.

"Thank you," I respond gratefully. "Thank you." At last. Two words to restore my wilting confidence. "Good job." Finally, Dr. Terence has acknowledged my daring (to me) medical decision. I begin to gush with explanation: "I think he met all the indications for a thoracotomy but I don't know if I can bring him back. He had vital signs in the field and arrested only a few minutes ago. Clearly it's because — "

"The king at the tomb in the dark," Dr. Terence interrupts, ignoring me. "Very dramatic. Good job. Loved it. Yes, I enjoyed that one."

As I realize that Dr. Terence is praising a theatrical product I created seven years previously and is at best indifferent to my present medical performance, the sweat begins to spread to the back of my neck.

Squeeze-release. Nothing.

"Are you satisfied, Thomas Becket?" I think to myself. Pride before the fall. Squeeze-release. Nothing.

Every once in a while I stop to confirm my failure. I feel the stillness of the heart for a few moments before starting again to squeeze-release, squeeze-release.

"Four minutes," the nurse announces.

"Pupils?" I ask.

The respiratory therapist opens the patient's eyelids and checks. "Fixed and dilated," she confirms.

I feel quite simply, and in spite of the half dozen allies all working this case with me, alone.

Inside my patient's chest my hands continue to work. Squeeze-release, squeeze-release.

And then . . . a quiver. A quiver. Molecules of sodium, potassium, and calcium have silently danced across membrane boundaries creating an electrical charge that had awakened tiny muscle fibers all over the heart. The tips of my fingers feel or perhaps only sense . . . a quiver.

"Yes, I enjoyed that one. Very much so," Dr. Terence continues, oblivious to the sea change that is taking place in the heart that I hold in my hand.

I'm more astonished than pleased. I'm feeling life restart itself. My hand now has a partner in a dance. I squeeze. It squeezes.

"We have a rhythm," the nurse says. Without emotion.

The heart was dancing in my hand. Not disorganized, but a steady, assured, confident dance, a two-step with a firm beat. I'm amazed.

Like an early morning bird, the "beep beep" of the heart monitor begins to chirp. With my left hand I take control of the rod compressing the aorta and slowly remove it, allowing blood to flow to the lower reaches of the body. I check the pressure monitor. Blood pressure is holding and beginning to climb.

"Pupils?" I ask.

"Responsive," the respiratory therapist reports. "Equal and reactive to light."

What a beautiful phrase: "Equal and reactive to light."

"Blood pressure 110 over 50," the nurse announces. His blood pressure has returned to near normal.

"Let's slow down the fluids and get him ready for transfer to the OR," I respond from somewhere.

I turn to Dr. Terence, still sweating. Me. Not him.

"Are you doing any more directing?" he pleasantly inquires.

Not right at this moment. I've been busy. Have you noticed? Busy.

"Not right now," I reply to Dr. Terence.

"Surgery's ready, Dr. Terence," the nurse calls. "Neurosurgery's already there."

I look down and realize that my right hand is still inside my patient's chest. His heart is beating strongly against my open palm. For a moment I regret that I have to take my hand out of his chest. It has become a magical place.

I arrange moist towels over the wound that I have made and stand watching as the nurses, one holding the metal arrow that still protrudes from the patient's neck, wheel my patient to the operating room.

"Thank you," I call. To no one in particular.

"Thank you," Dr. Terence replies with an easy smile as he disappears around a corner and out of the ER. The cubicle is suddenly ordinary: empty, used, and messy. I take a breath and try to refocus, to end my connection with *my* patient, a patient that has suddenly been abducted from my care.

After a few moments, I take off my gloves and go to wash my hands.

"Nice work, Doctor," someone calls from over my shoulder. It's one of the paramedics, the one I had talked to on the radio. The paramedics had stayed to watch.

"That patient could not have been better treated at any hospital. Anywhere."

"Well, thank you." The praise is a complete surprise. "You, too. It worked, didn't it? Thank you." I'm still adrenalized and feel as if I'm not making complete sense.

"Impressive. It was an honor to work with you," the paramedic adds on his way out to the ambulance.

"You, too. You, too." I don't know what else to say. And I don't really feel like talking.

For five hours a vascular surgeon worked to repair the neck vessels that had been lacerated by the metal rod. A neurosurgeon worked to remove the rod from the spinal column in which it was embedded. The vertebral arteries along the spinal column had been cut. They could not be repaired. After five hours my patient bled again. This time to death.

Although I held his heart in my hand, I didn't know much about him until his funeral was announced four days later in the newspaper. That's when I learned how hard he had worked, often putting in extra hours on the weekend. I was surprised also to discover that his wife was a nurse in the hospital and that she was at work two floors above me when I was trying to save her husband's life.

Two weeks later I return to the same emergency department. I'm no longer a resident. I'm complete. I don't strut but I do take up some extra space and time wandering the momentarily quiet ER in the hope that someone there has seen my "special" case. The case that still amazes me and angers me at the same time. So close. So close.

I walk slowly past the nurses' station. The paramedics in the ER that morning are not the same ones with whom I had worked. I pick up a chart and stroll to see my first patient of the day.

"What can I do for you?" I ask.

"My toes," he says.

"Yes?" I respond with a smile. His toes look fine. No infection or signs of trauma. His toenails, on the other hand, are a mess.

"My toenails," he specifies.

"Yes?" I try to sound reassuring. They were definitely *his* toenails. Overgrown, long, and dirty.

"They need cutting," he observes, pleasantly. "I have trouble bending over. And I have a tremor."

"Uh-huh." I've caught the "uh-huh" disease.

"That's why I'm here. So you can cut them."

"You came to the emergency department to get your toenails cut?" I ask in disbelief.

"Yes. They're way too long."

I have to agree with that.

I look around the cubicle and smile. It's the same cubicle in which I stood two weeks earlier proudly holding a new-beating heart. I get up and open a wooden drawer along the wall. Searching through screwdrivers, tape, metal cutters, and clamps, I find a pair of oversized toenail clippers. I sit down on a small metal stool, hold his toes in my hand, and clip.

BRUTE

BY *Richard Selzer, M.D.*

You must never again set your anger upon a patient. You were tired, you said, and therefore it happened. Now that you have excused yourself, there is no need for me to do it for you.

Imagine that you yourself go to a doctor because you have chest pain. You are worried that there is something the matter with your heart. Chest pain is your Chief Complaint. It happens that your doctor has been awake all night with a patient who has been bleeding from a peptic ulcer of his stomach. He is tired. That is your doctor's Chief Complaint. I have chest pain, you tell him. I am tired, he says.

Still I confess to some sympathy for you. I know what tired is.

Listen: It is twenty-five years ago in the Emergency Room. It is two o'clock in the morning. There has been a day and night of stabbings, heart attacks and automobile accidents. A commotion at the door: A huge black man is escorted by four policemen into the Emergency Room. He is handcuffed. At the door, the man rears as though to shake off the men who cling to his arms and press him from the rear. Across the full length of his forehead is a laceration. It is deep to the bone. I know it without probing its depths. The split of his black flesh is like the white wound of an ax in the trunk of a tree. Again and again he throws his head and shoulders forward, then back, rearing, roaring. The policemen ride him like parasites. Had he horns he would gore them. Blind and trussed, the man shakes them about, rattles them. But if one of them loses his grip, the others are still fixed and sucking. The man is hugely drunk — toxic, fuming, murderous — a great mythic beast broken loose in the city, surprised in his night raid by a phalanx of legionnaires armed with clubs and revolvers.

I do not know the blow that struck him on the brow. Or was there any blow? Here is a brow that might have burst on its own, spilling out its excess of rage, bleeding itself toward ease. Perhaps it was done by a jealous lover, a woman, or a man who will not pay him the ten dollars he won in a bet, or still another who has hurled the one insult that he cannot bear to hear. Perhaps it was done by the police themselves. From the distance of many years and from the safety of my little study, I choose to see it thus:

The helmeted corps rounds the street corner. A shout. "There he is!" And they clatter toward him. He stands there for a moment, lurching. Something upon which he had been feeding falls from his open mouth. He turns to face the policemen. For him it is not a new challenge. He is scarred as a Zulu from his many battles. Almost from habit he ascends to the combat. One or more of them falls under his flailing arms until — there is the swing of a truncheon, a sound as though a melon has been dropped from a great height. The white wedge appears upon the seating brow of the black man, a waving fall of blood pours across eyes and cheeks.

The man is blinded by it; he is stunned. Still he reaches forth to make contact with the enemy, to do one more piece of damage. More blows to the back, the chest and again to the face. Bloody spume flies from his head as lifted by a great wind. The police are spattered with it. They stare at each other with an abstract horror and disgust. One last blow, and blind as Samson, the black man undulates, rolling in a splayfooted circle. But he does not go down. The police are upon him then, pinning him, cuffing his wrists, kneeing him toward the van. Through the back window of the wagon — a netted panther.

In the Emergency Room he is led to the treatment area and to me. There is a vast dignity about him. He keeps his own counsel. What is he thinking? I wonder. The police urge him up on the table. They put him down. They restrain his arms with straps. I examine the wound, and my heart sinks. It is twelve centimeters long, irregular, jagged and, as I knew, to the skull. It will take at least two hours.

I am tired. Also to the bone. But something else . . . Oh, let me not deny it. I am ravished by the sight of him, the raw, untreated flesh, his very wildness which suggests less a human than a great and beautiful animal. As though by the addition of the wound, his body is more than it was, more of a body. I begin to cleanse and debride the wound. At my touch, he stirs and groans. "Lie still," I tell him. But now he rolls his head from side to side so that I cannot work. Again and again he lifts his pelvis from the table, strains against his bonds, then falls heavily. He roars something, not quite language. "Hold still," I say. "I cannot stitch your forehead unless you hold still."

Perhaps it is the petulance in my voice that makes him resume his struggle against all odds to be free. Perhaps he understands that it is only a cold, thin official voice such as mine, and not the billy clubs of half-a-dozen cops that can rob him of his dignity. And so he strains and screams. But why can he not sense that I am tired? He spits and curses and rolls his head to escape from my fingers. It is quarter to three in the morning. I have not yet begun to stitch. I lean close to him; his steam fills my nostrils. "Hold still," I say.

"*You* fuckin' hold still," he says to me in a clear, fierce voice. Suddenly, I am in the fury with him. Somehow he has managed to capture me, to pull me inside his cage. Now we are two brutes hissing and battling at each other. But I do not fight fairly.

I go to the cupboard and get from it two packets of heavy, braided silk suture and a large curved needle. I pass one of the heavy silk sutures through the eye of the needle. I take the needle in the jaws of a needle holder, and I pass the needle through the mattress of the stretcher. And I tie the thread tightly so that his head is pulled to the right. I do exactly the same to his left earlobe, and again I tie the thread tightly so that his head is facing directly upward.

"I have sewn your ears to the stretcher," I say. "Move, and you'll rip 'em off." And leaning close I say in a whisper, "Now *you* fuckin' hold still."

I do more. I wipe the gelatinous clots from his eyes so that he can see. And I lean over him from the head of the table, so that my face is directly above his, upside down. And I grin. It is the cruelest grin of my life. Torturers must grin like that, beheaders and operators of racks.

But now he does hold still. Surely it is not just fear of tearing his earlobes. He is too deep into his passion for that. It is more likely some beastly wisdom that tells him that at last he has no hope of winning. That it is time to cut his losses, to slink off into high grass. Or is it some sober thought that pierces his wild brain, lacerating him in such a way that a hundred nightsticks could not? The thought of a woman who is waiting for him, perhaps? Or a child who, the next day and the week after that, will stare up at his terrible scars with a silent wonder that will shame him? For whatever reason, he is perfectly still.

It is four o'clock in the morning as I take the first stitch in his wound. At five-thirty, I snip each of the silks in his earlobes. He is released from his leg restrainers and pulled to a sitting position. The bandage on his head is a white turban. A single drop of blood in each earlobe, like a ruby. He is a maharajah.

Brute

45

The police return. All this time they have been drinking coffee with the nurses, the orderlies, other policemen, whomever. For over three hours the man and I have been alone in our devotion to the wound. "I have finished," I tell them. Roughly, they haul him from the stretcher and prod him toward the door. "Easy, easy," I call after them. And, to myself, if you hit him again . . .

Even now, so many years later, this ancient rage of mine returns to peck among my dreams. I have only to close my eyes to see him again wielding his head and jaws, to hear once more those words at which the whole of his trussed body came hurtling toward me. How sorry I will always be. Not being able to make it up to him for that grin.

DEATH BY CHOCOLATE

BY *Hamish MacLaren, M.D.*

Every so often, a patient will attempt to work one over on us, to pull a fast one. Perhaps he will acquire documentation from the ER for an accident that never happened, or he might attempt to steal the television set from the waiting room. Anything not chained down is fair game — patients' belongings, prescription pads, even pieces of medical equipment that you would have thought had no use to anyone outside of medicine: blood pressure cuffs, pulse oximeters, cardiac monitors. And of course, some patients come to the ER with the intention of receiving medication, particularly intravenous narcotics, for spurious ailments. Commonly such patients will be able to recount the classic symptoms for, say, renal colic. When called upon to do so, they will produce, by covert means, a sample of urine containing blood, which will appear to confirm the diagnosis of a stone in the renal tract. Such patients are conventionally treated by Demerol injection. This is, in fact, the outcome that they seek. Shortly after receiving the medication, they are found to have left without having been discharged, and are unlikely to return. Their next presentation will be in another hospital emergency room, under another name.

The first time this ever happened to me — I should say the first time I became *aware* that a patient had tricked me in this way — I was furious. I allowed myself a short but passionate tantrum during which I jumped up and down, snarled, kicked doors, and harangued a patient who had, of course, long since left. But why was I so angry? Was it not, after all, merely a dent in the *amour propre?* Nobody likes to be made a fool of. Suppose I'd discovered my patient's little game before he had received his injection. Would it have made any difference? Would I have been able to alter his long-term behavior significantly? Probably not. Therefore all I was really squealing about was the improper use of one vial of Demerol. As a matter of fact, the only real loser was the patient himself. Nowadays I console myself with such thoughts when taken advantage of in this way.

But the trick young Tracy pulled off was much more subtle than the old drop-of-blood-in-the-urine trick. Its desired outcome was certainly more bizarre, and when I eventually realized that I had been gulled, I must say I didn't really snarl. In fact, I would have laughed had I not gagged.

It was eleven o'clock at night when Tracy arrived, with two of her friends. They were school friends, all fifteen years old. They had, they informed me, been out to dinner. All three wore short black numbers, and they had been rather heavy-handed with the application of makeup. Under the garish strip lighting of the reception area, this made them look younger, not the intended older, than they really were. Tracy was thin. She had long red hair, which tonight she wore up. She wore red lipstick and rouged cheeks, but it was clear that beneath the makeup and the freckles her skin was pale. I guessed she was about ninety pounds. They were in strained conversation with the triage nurse when I first spotted them. There was a kind of woman-to-woman resentment, a caustic frisson, in the air. After all, they had come to see a doctor, and why was this nurse bombarding them with questions?

Chris Bailey, who was doing triage for the night, eventually turned to me. She raised her eyes momentarily to the ceiling. "Tylenol overdose. Sounds like quite a big one, about an hour ago."

Tracy was popped onto a gurney and wheeled into Resuscitation. Thus she assumed the sick role, even though people who ingest toxic doses of Tylenol seldom become unwell in the early stages. It is later, at about seventy-two hours, that they become sick. By this time, the liver damage is irreversible, jaundice grows deep, and the patient vomits, and vomits, and vomits. Renal failure follows liver failure. We monitor the astronomically high blood levels of spilled liver enzymes, and thus preside over the patient's demise with all the ritual uselessness of high priests.

People who overdose on drugs for one reason or another are often uncommunicative, but Tracy was blithesome enough.

"How much Tylenol did you take, Tracy?"

She had intelligent eyes. "Lots!"

"And when did you take them?"

She looked at her friends. "What time, Charlie?" (I thought, Charlie? Funny name for a girl. Must be Charlotte, or Charmaine. Or maybe Charlene.)

"Just about an hour ago, I guess," said Charlie. "It was just after dessert."

They all giggled.

What was so funny about dessert?

"Remember, you went to the ladies' room," said the third girl. She spoke in a low voice, almost conspiratorial. Half of her face was concealed behind long hair, and she avoided eye contact. "You went to the bathroom while we ordered coffee."

"Special coffee," chipped in Charlie.

"And when you came back you said you'd done it."

Chris Bailey came through the door. She was bearing Tracy's handbag and a dozen blister packs of acetaminophen tablets. She had been rummaging. The three girls scowled at her.

"Twelve packs," said Chris.

"Did you take them all, Tracy?"

She nodded, with an "aren't I a clever girl?" expression. I made a calculation. One hundred and forty-four 500-milligram tablets; 72 grams of Tylenol in a decidedly underweight adolescent girl. Certainly a lethal dose, but as we were seeing her one hour post ingestion, we had plenty of time. How on earth could somebody swallow 144 pills without throwing up? And after dinner, too?

I asked her, "And why did you take them?"

Tracy looked at her friends and bit her lip. I had the vague feeling she was trying not to laugh, and also that she was recounting something that had already been said in rehearsal.

"My uncle raped me." There was a pause.

". . . when I was seven." They all exploded into a gale of laughter. Tracy was the first to stop laughing. She gave her friends a warning look, whispered, "Shut up!" and then said to me, "Okay, sorry. Actually, I've just fallen out with my boyfriend." I had the feeling that Charlie was having difficulty suppressing her laughter, but Tracy was now firmly in control. She looked serious.

"Look. I'm really sorry. I know it was silly of me, and I'm really sorry to be wasting your time like this. You must get really sick of people like me."

I said, "Occasionally."

"Brent and I broke up this afternoon." (I thought to myself, Yes, it would have to be a Brent, or a Jason, or a Darryl.) "Charlie and Donna, here, took me out to dinner to cheer me up, and I thought I was going to be okay. Then, I don't know, something came over me." Two huge tears gathered in Tracy's eyes and spilled down her cheeks. Charlie put an arm around her and said, "Come on, Trace. Brent's not worth it." I had the impression that Tracy was a very clever girl, that she could switch any expression onto her face, that she could be lachrymose at will.

She sniffled into a tissue. "I wasn't trying to — to kill myself or anything like that."

"You're having a bloody good try."

So she switched off tears and sadness and switched on fear and alarm.

"Really? I'll be okay, won't I?"

"You'll be okay if we wash your stomach out."

"Oh, God. Do I have to?"

"Absolutely."

"What happens if I don't?"

"You get very sick."

She fixed me with her wide, appraising, intelligent eyes. "Would I die?"

"Probably."

She absorbed this piece of information. Charlie said, "Come on, Trace, you'd better let them do it."

She nodded, mutely. I said to Chris Bailey, "Could you set up for a gastric lavage, Chris, and we'll give fifty grams of charcoal. I'll take some blood. We'll check a Tylenol and aspirin level." I said to Tracy, "Your parents at home?"

"Mom is. Dad's in Australia."

"We'd better call her and tell her what's going on. Okay?"

She nodded. She was back in tearful mode again. "I've been such an idiot. I really didn't mean to. I don't know what it was. Cry for help, I suppose."

If there is one threadbare cliché in the whole gamut of populist soap opera medicine that is guaranteed to grate on me, it is "cry for help." Cry for help indeed! More like a coolly premeditated act of manipulation designed to bring about a desired piece of behavior on the part of some relative, friend, or lover. So who was it? The absent Brent? Who was being manipulated?

I should have delved more deeply into the morass of Tracy's unutterably complex psyche, but I didn't have the time, and, to be perfectly honest, I didn't have the interest. I could have spent all night chatting with Tracy about the underlying causes of her plight and she would keep on spilling the beans, but at best it would all be a hygienic, sanitized, cosmetically acceptable version of the truth. I could peel off layer after layer of the onion and never find a core. I didn't have the skill that I had sometimes observed in a really talented psychiatrist, to take in and analyze all the carefully censored data that patients chose to present, and to undercut it, to scythe through it all with a devastating, cripplingly hurtful comment, after which the patient, rendered naked, would tell the truth for the first time. But I knew Tracy would dance circles round me and I would never discover her hidden agenda. Besides, there was good reason for cracking on and emptying her stomach of all that Tylenol before she absorbed much more of it.

Chris had set up the tray with the length of plastic tubing and a stout steel funnel to fit on the end, large pitchers of water transformed into normal saline by the addition of a measured quantity of sodium chloride; a bucket to catch the gastric aspirate, K-Y jelly to lubricate the tube. Most of what we needed was there.

I said to Tracy, "Have you ever had this done before?"

"Good God, no! What do you take me for?" It was a question I might have answered, but I didn't.

"Okay, let me talk you through this. It's a little uncomfortable." That, I reflected, was the understatement of the year. I gag easily, and if I ever had the misfortune to be subjected to this procedure, I'm sure I would require six burly orderlies to hold me down. "Just concentrate on your breathing," I said. "We use the suction line here to make sure you don't choke, so you'll be just fine." I picked up the triangular wooden mouthpiece and wrapped gauze around it.

"This is something for you to bite on, so you don't bite the tube. Do you have any false teeth?"

"Fuck off!"

Chris was saying to Charlie, "Probably best for you to wait in the waiting room. It's not the most pleasant procedure to watch."

Tracy exclaimed, and it was almost inarticulate because the mouthpiece was now in place, "Charlie stays!"

Charlie said, "I'll be okay."

I nodded. "Fair enough. Would you like to hold Tracy's hands? Keep them down, away from the tube." She did so.

"Tracy, we're just going to tip the bed a little head down now. It helps with the wash-out. Suction ready, Chris?" I applied a little more K-Y to the tube. "Okay. Off we go. Swallow the tube now." It passed easily. There was a cough and a gasp and an inarticulate gulp of protest. "Very good, Tracy! The tube's down, the worst part's over. Remember about the breathing. Concentrate on the breathing." She settled down. There wasn't going to be a problem, she wasn't going to panic.

I emptied a liter of normal saline into a jug and tested it for temperature. It was tepid. I poured about 100 milliliters into the funnel and raised it, with the tube toward the ceiling. The water flowed easily. I lowered the funnel to the bucket on the floor. I suddenly realized I'd forgotten to put on a plastic gown. Oh, well. I hoped it was not going to be a messy one. The patient was relaxed, and there was no coughing. I'd intubated the right aperture. That was always good to know! I poured about 250 milliliters into the funnel. Up to the ceiling, down to the floor; the fluid flowed easily but only a trace of it was coming out, and no gastric content. Another 250 milliliters, up, and down. Only 50 milliliters came back. I laid a hand on Tracy's abdomen. It was distended. I thought, Well, there's a three-course dinner in there and a ton of Tylenol. We should get *something* back.

"All right, Trace?"

"Argh!"

"Good."

I pressed on the abdomen. "Just a little gentle massage to get things moving."

I said to Charlie, "What restaurant were you in?"

"Death by Chocolate."

"Death by *what?*"

"Chocolate."

"What on earth is that?"

"It's a dessert restaurant, on the waterfront, along Tamaki Drive. They specialize in chocolate puddings."

"Sounds pretty revolting to me. So you just had dessert there?"

"No, we had a three-course meal."

"I see. They actually serve wholesome, nourishing food as well?"

"No. Now, let's see, for an appetizer I had Wicked Willy's Sexy Sundae: chocolate croutons with whipped double cream layered in a liaison of fudge and marzipan. Then for the main entree, Caramel Bavarois in whorls of toffeed creamy eclair, festooned in a dew of almond truffle and topped by a riot of praline, solid milk, and Mississippi Mud . . ."

I have long been fascinated, in a sick way, with the 46XX obsession with the dessert cart. Just as, of all the Seven Deadly Sins, the cafard, hamartia, and nemesis for the male is Lust, so, the female of the species seems to be tempted, seduced, and finally ruined by Gluttony. And indeed, from the viewpoint of the male, it almost seems that female gluttony is a kind of lust. I have come to dread that moment in a restaurant, particularly if one is dining with an attractive woman for the first time, when the dessert cart is wheeled laboriously across. Perhaps it is, in me, the wretched jealousy of a jilted lover. Is there anything more demeaning than the thought of being abandoned for a brandy snap, of playing cuckold to a pastry? It wouldn't be so bad if this lovely dining companion chose the fattest and creamiest pudding on the deck and proceeded to consume it with silent and concentrated greed. What is unendurable is the protracted verbal foreplay preceding the cuisine's devouring, the knowing looks exchanged between the girl and the waiter as if they were both party to some delightfully salacious conspiracy, the crescendo of ecstasy as each culinary delight is revealed on the various levels of the cart and then, worst of all, the feigned hypocritical show of reluctance — "Oh, I mustn't . . . oh, I shouldn't . . . ooooooh . . ."

"Stop!" I said to Charlie. "Don't tell me any more." I poured 400 milliliters of normal saline into the funnel and raised it to the ceiling. Yet I just had to ask.

"And what did Tracy have?"

"Oh, she had Death by Chocolate."

"Ah. No doubt, the chef's pièce de résistance."

"Mmm. Yummy. For two people — except, she wasn't sharing."

"Was that her appetizer or main course?" I pushed the distended abdomen again.

"She ate three in a row."

And at that moment, as if in confirmation of this remarkable feat, a curious substance began, slowly but inexorably, to emerge through the gastric lavage tube. A dark, intense, sticky brown goo. Too intense, and too sticky, for the tube. Suddenly there was a great abdominal heave and the entire gastric contents bypassed the tube in her mouth. A great projectile wall of mud engulfed me. The room was suffused in the aroma of sugary toffee, tinged with the vaguely acidic reminiscence of Parmesan cheese. Ruefully I reflected once again that I'd omitted to put on a plastic gown. I stuck the base of my tongue against the roof of my mouth, closed my mind to the horror of Death by Chocolate, and continued with the lavage. No sign of any tablet material, I observed forlornly. Now the lavage fluid flowed in and out easily, gradually changing color from dark brown, to pale tan, then the color of an elegant Chardonnay, and finally, crystal clear. I muttered to Chris, "Charcoal." The charcoal looked even more evil than the chocolate, black and thick, but it flowed easily down the tube. A little saline chaser, and then I grasped the tube at Tracy's mouth and put a kink in it.

"Cough!"

And as she did so I smoothly extracted the lavage tube. Not smoothly enough. She heaved and gagged, and the charcoal returned, messily. Chris readjusted the position of the gurney, removed the mouth guard, and wiped some chocolate/charcoal from Tracy's face. I surveyed the room. It was a bomb site. Six feet away on the wall, tiny flecks of black and brown rose to above eye level.

I said, equably, "Tracy, would you consider yourself to be a sensible eater?" I began to take more conscious account of her weight, of her lack of subcutaneous substance, of the fact that I could visually count all her ribs, right down to the twelfth. She said, hopefully, "I eat a lot of salads." Charlie was shaking her head. "She chucks, Doctor."

"She vomits?"

Charlie nodded. "Binges and chucks. That's what I thought she was doing in the john tonight."

A staff nurse opened the door and passed a sheet of paper across to Chris. It was a faxed result from the laboratory. Chris glanced at it.

"Tylenol level — ZERO."

I had thought that the absent Brent, Tracy's ex, was the fall guy in her little game. But it was I who was the patsy. I said to her, "Tracy, you've just taken me for a ride."

TOUGH LOVE

BY *Pamela Grim, M.D.*

Now, here's one for you." I looked up from the chart I was writing on. There were two police officers, both big guys, each flanking a reedy young man, boy really, dressed in shabby clothes. He stood blinking, molelike, in the bright light of the ER.

"Who, what?" Bill, the evening charge nurse, asked. He was sitting next to me. We were having a terrible day. Two unsuccessful resuscitations before nine A.M. and since, we had been working frantically to catch up. This was an inner-city ER. The patients were a grab bag of trauma, critical cardiac cases, drug overdoses, and the like, all mixed in with sprained ankles and sore throats.

One of the officers lifted up a paper bag and shook it.

"We got called by this kid's parents. They said he was acting goofy, high on drugs or something. So we went out and we found him with *this*."

Bill peered over the top of his glasses. "Okay," he said. "What is *this?*"

"*This,*" the officer said, shaking the bag again, "is a hamster."

Bill nodded. "Of course, a hamster."

"Not just a hamster. A *dead* hamster."

Bill pushed his glasses back in place, waiting for the payoff. "Uh-huh," he said.

The second officer leaned forward. "He had it in his mouth."

I had gone back to charting, not really listening closely, but at this point I stopped and looked up at the boy. Bill didn't even skip a beat. "Did he say why?"

"Because it was dead," the boy said suddenly and then, as if he had startled himself, he backed a few steps away and resumed staring down at his shabby sneakers. He mumbled something I couldn't hear.

"What?" I said, sitting forward.

"Randell," the second police officer said and looked back at him. "Randell, tell the doctor what you told us."

Scarcely audible, Randell said, "CPR."

"CPR?"

"Yeah," Officer Number One said. "He told us that he was trying to perform CPR on the hamster. That's why he had it in his mouth."

"And," Officer Number Two said, not to be outdone, "not only that, he was doing all this in the garage and he had the car hood up and the battery out of the car and he had — "

" — he had some stereo wires hooked up to the battery and was trying to shock the hamster," Officer Number One broke in. "You know, defibrillate it — like the paramedics do on television. He said it was the only way to save the hamster's life."

"Rocky's life," the boy said. "The hamster's name is Rocky. *Was* Rocky."

"That's when his parents called us," Officer Number Two said, putting the bag down on the desk and raising his hands. "What were we going to do? Arrest him for attempted hamster resuscitation?"

Bill looked directly at the boy. "You tried to defibrillate a hamster?"

The boy kept looking down at his feet but he nodded, cleared his throat, and took a deep breath. "It seemed to make sense at the time" was all he said.

His parents showed up a half hour later. I still hadn't had a chance to get in to see the boy. All I knew was that he was seventeen, older than he looked. The parents were well dressed, in fact, very well dressed. They obviously came from a well-to-do neighborhood out of the usual service area of our ER (except when the police were involved). They kept glancing around nervously with an obvious distaste, tinged here and there with fear, at the usual ER bad news crowd. A woman sat next to them holding some bloody gauze to her head. She was a prostitute who had suffered a scalp laceration when beaten up by her pimp. Passing by were a couple of men on stretchers, fully immobilized on wooden backboards and neck braces, borne along by paramedics. On the other side of me there were the gurneys where a couple of drunks were sleeping it off — the gurneys were in the hallway because we had nowhere else to put them.

The father, looking around at all this, finally spotted me and led his wife over to the desk. He was wearing a well-cut suit and a tie with a diagonal pattern that, close up, revealed itself to be made of tiny sailboats, blue spinnakers billowing. He had obviously just come from work. A lawyer, I guessed; even his haircut looked expensive. The boy's mother was a tall, slender woman, elaborately coiffed, carrying an expensive leather handbag. "Socialite," I thought. The father started to introduce himself to me when he was momentarily distracted by Bill, who was sitting next to me, giving report on the phone. Bill looked the way he always looked: hair tied back in a ponytail, large hoop earrings, a straggly goatee, dark glasses, and a badge on his scrub top that read, "So many doctors, so few bullets." The father shook his head slowly and turned to me. At least I had a white coat on.

I introduced myself and shook the clammy, limp hand of the mother. They were the "D's." I took them over to a quiet corner so we could hear each other. "So . . ." I said. "What's been going on?"

"I think it's drugs," Mr. D said. "I don't know where he's getting them from but I think it's drugs."

"He's never touched drugs," Mrs. D said vehemently in turn. "I don't know how you can think that."

"How else do you explain all this?" Mr. D whispered fiercely to Mrs. D.

"I can't," Mrs. D replied, equally fiercely. "But there has to be an answer." She stood there, tight-lipped, ashen-faced. Obviously these two had been disagreeing about their son for years. They each looked off in a different direction, both looking equally anxious and bewildered.

"Tell me what the problems have been," I said.

Mrs. D groped for words. I could see she was not accustomed to sharing details from family life with a stranger, even if the stranger was a doctor. But, now, the situation had become desperate. "Last week he borrowed the car. Stole it really. He got the keys out of my purse, and . . . and . . . went out joyriding. He ended up smashing it against a freeway barricade. A thousand dollars' worth of damage, and he could have been killed. I couldn't believe it. He knew he wasn't supposed to have been driving the car."

"He's always been more or less of a discipline problem," Mr. D added. Now that the ice was broken, everything started tumbling out. "I think, basically, he's a good kid," he added softly, "but he's so damn irresponsible, never listens. We finally took him to see a psychologist last year and the psychologist did all these tests and said he had — What is it he's supposed to have?" Mr. D, frowning, forehead furrowed, turned to Mrs. D.

"Attention deficit disorder."

"Right, attention deficit disorder. Which makes sense to me in a way. Randell has never been able to pay attention. He can't finish anything he starts; he gets distracted by anything, everything, and it's just been getting worse."

Mrs. D broke in. "The school psychologist said he was learning disabled. Or dyslexic. I'm not sure what the difference between the two of them is. She said that this is why Randell does so poorly in school when he's so very bright on his test scores and everything." She literally wrung her hands in front of me; the tissue in her hands was in tatters. Mr. D stared off into space. He looked infinitely sad.

"About the hamster," I said.

"He's a bright boy," Mr. D said. "He knows everything there is to know about taking a bicycle apart and putting it back together. He spends hours and hours in the garage."

"The hamster . . ." I said again.

"Rocky? Oh, he's had that old hamster for years." Mr. D sighed, still absorbed with his worries about Randell. "He never seems to learn from experience, no matter how often he screws up. I feel like I'm at the end of my rope with him. He isn't attending classes at school; I'm sure he's going to flunk several courses this year. He stays out until three in the morning, no matter what we say. Or he doesn't come home at all. I don't know where he is half the time."

"He's impulsive," his mother added. "And he fidgets. He fidgeted when he was little and he never grew out of it."

"Diet therapy," Mr. D said meditatively. "People have suggested diet therapy because sometimes this disorder is caused by, you know, allergies, like allergies to wheat or to nylon. I don't know, that seemed a little wacky to me."

"I guess we spoiled him. He's our youngest. We never went through anything like this with our other children." Mrs. D paused and took a deep breath. "The school psychologist says that a big part of the problem is that Randell has absolutely no self-esteem."

Mr. D broke in. "I think he's basically a discipline problem. He has no idea of the consequences of his actions." Mr. D stared moodily down at his hands. "How can you give your child everything you have and he still ends up with no self-esteem?"

"I understand," I said, though I was lying. I was sure I didn't understand any more than they did.

"We've been so desperate," Mrs. D said. "Nobody can give us any answers, so a couple of months ago we went to this seminar on Tough Love."

"I'm sorry," I said. "On what?"

"Tough Love. It's a course on how to . . . well, I guess they say . . . 'set limits' . . . on your children." She reached into her handbag and brought out a hardcover book.

She showed it to me. *Tough Love, or Raising Children in a Modern Age.* A picture of the author, I presume, stared up at us from the cover. We all three stood there looking down at her, nodding our heads, as if maybe she did have some answers.

A patient came in with pulmonary edema. I rushed off and couldn't get back to the D's for an hour, at least. I finally found them waiting in the pelvic room, the only room we had left to put them in. The boy was sitting on the examining table, legs dangling between the stirrups. Despite the heat outside, he wore a T-shirt, two unbuttoned shirts, and a jacket. His parents sat off to the side, arms folded stiffly, mother with her purse in her lap. No one was talking. The boy was pale, gray even. He coughed a phlegmy smoker's cough, like an old man, and stared down at his feet.

I had his chart in my hands. "Randell, is it? Hi, Randell. I'm the doctor on today."

"Oh," Randell said. He looked up at me skeptically but said nothing. He returned his gaze to his sneakers and just sat there.

"Randell, honey," his mother said. "Talk to the doctor for us, won't you?"

The boy said nothing.

"Randell," I said, as gently as I could. "What was this about you stealing the car?"

Randell shrugged his shoulders, head down, lips moving — but soundlessly. Then he mumbled something.

"What? What did you say?"

"My parents wouldn't let me drive the car."

Mr. D broke in. "He lost his privileges to use the car because of his grades. When he brings his grades up he can use the car."

"Randell . . . ," I said. "How do you feel about that?"

Randell shrugged again. "It's okay."

"Then why did you steal it?" his father asked.

Randell shook his head. "It's hard to explain."

"Well, try."

The boy looked up suddenly at his father. "I wasn't supposed to drive it. I knew that. I was confused. I wrecked it."

"Randell," he said, leaning forward. "Are you doing drugs?"

Randell thought a moment, as if he was trying to remember. "Marijuana," he said finally.

"Lately?" I asked.

Randell thought again. "No, not for a while."

"Randell," I said and pulled my chair up close. I was looking up to him where he sat, the least threatening position I could find. "Randell, did you kill your hamster?"

Randell looked up at the ceiling. "You mean Rocky?" He paused for a moment and looked down at me. He slowly nodded his head. "Yup," he said.

"Why?"

Randell shrugged and looked away from me. Finally he said, "It's a secret."

"Why is it a secret?"

"Because of what happened."

"Tell me," I said.

He leaned his head from side to side, deliberating. "Rocky is dead because I killed him. I killed him because he was dead. His name is Rocket J. Squirrel, but he's not a squirrel. He's a hamster." Randell lifted up his hands and stared at them for a moment, then he looked at me. "I broke his neck."

"Why would you do something like that?" his mother asked from behind me.

Randell shrugged and looked away. Finally he said, "So I wouldn't kill my father."

I heard a sharp intake of breath behind me and a sigh. I leaned forward even more and put my hand gently on Randell's knee. I was pretty sure what was coming.

"Have you been thinking about killing your father?"

The boy shrugged, and then said, "Yup."

"How long?"

"Since the car. Since he wouldn't let me . . . maybe before. I don't know. I think about it a lot. I don't think it's normal to think that." He looked up at me. "Do you think it's normal to think that?"

"Randell," I said. "Have you been hearing voices?"

He looked at me as if I had guessed a secret he thought had been perfectly hidden. "Huh?" he said. He squinted at me.

"You know, people talking to you who don't seem to be really there."

"Oh," Randell said, and stared back down at his shoes. "I'm not sure," he said.

"How do you mean, you're 'not sure'? "

"Well" — he cleared his throat and took a deep breath — "actually, you have to understand, it's about the sewer system."

"What about the sewer system?"

"It's underneath me."

"The sewer system?"

"Yes, and there's a force in the sewer system that's run by nuclear power." He looked up at his parents as if this would explain everything. "Don't tell anyone else but it's tracking my thoughts. I shouldn't even be talking to you because it's actually spying on everything I say." Randell looked almost relieved as he said all this, as if the strain of keeping this a secret had finally been too much for him. "I don't like being here with you. When you talk to me it's like you are joining forces with them." He sighed. "I'm sorry, but, really." He studied his sneakers as he spoke. "The sewer system is taking over my body and making me extinct." He sighed.

Randell looked bright somehow. He seemed almost happy to be sharing this world at last, this strange peculiar world he secretly inhabited.

I turned around and caught a glimpse of Mrs. D. She had a hand raised to her mouth and was staring at her son as if she had just seen a monster arise from the abyss.

"I'm sorry about the car," Randell said. He was rocking back and forth. "I was just so confused in the head. I figured if I wrecked it, you know, killed the car, then I would end the confusion in my head." He looked up toward his parents and even leaned forward a little. He whispered in a stage whisper, loud enough for all of us to hear, "I'd like to go home. It's very difficult sitting around an emergency room watching yourself die."

He looked back down at his feet again and resumed rocking.

"What's the matter with him?"

They both rushed me, pulling me aside, clutching at my elbows. I had been called out of the room for another emergency that we had finally stabilized.

"Well," I said. I was writing on Randell's chart quickly so I could get him referred to Psychiatry. "It's not drugs." By now I had the drug screen results back, and they were negative — no drugs on board. "His urine is clean. We are going to need Psychiatry to evaluate him." I was trying to move them along; there were other, sicker patients. But when I looked up and caught a glimpse of Mrs. D's face, all frantic and fearful, I felt ashamed for trying to brush her off. Really, though, I told myself, I was not in a position to give them a diagnosis. That would take a psychiatrist and months of observation.

I looked at them again. How could I not tell these two frightened and bewildered people something that might allow them to make some sense of what was going on? How could I leave them hanging until we finally got a psychiatrist here, which could be hours?

"Well," I sighed, "I can tell you what I think it is."

"What?"

"People who talk like your son is talking now are often having their first psychotic break. It happens with schizophrenics."

The two of them both stood silently for a moment. I thought: In some way, they knew this already. Mr. D seemed to deflate a little, become smaller. He leaned against his wife.

"You mean like a split personality?" Mrs. D asked.

"It's not really that. The split is not in the person. The split is between the person and reality."

They both stared off in the direction of the drunks on the stretchers. Mrs. D's face was bunched, on the brink of crying. Her husband was virtually unreadable. Should I have said anything? Should I not have?

"Schizophrenia is a mental illness," Mr. D. said, finally summoning himself.

"That's right."

"Diagnosed by a psychiatrist."

"That's right."

"And you're not a psychiatrist."

"I'm not."

He nodded. I could see him weighing the evidence. "How does somebody treat schizophrenia?"

"Medication. A supportive environment."

"Supportive environment. You mean like a psychiatric hospital."

"Sometimes that's helpful."

Mrs. D was kneading her hands. "You don't grow out of schizophrenia . . . if you have schizophrenia."

"No, not usually."

She clutched her purse, staring out across the busy hallway. Finally she turned to me and touched my shoulder. "But he's going to be all right, isn't he? He is going to go back to normal eventually? Isn't he?"

"I don't know," I said. I didn't want to say what I was thinking, which was that someone with a first break at seventeen had a poor prognosis.

"He'll never be all right," she said. Two giant tears tinged with black mascara slipped out of the corner of each eye. "Never, never?"

"Shh," her husband said. He put his arm around her and pulled her gently over to the wall, out of the way of hallway traffic. He pulled her head down to his shoulder so she could cry in peace.

A baby howled in Room 9A. I heard it as I walked back to the nurses' station. I had a headache and, for some reason, this headache was associated with a mental image of Mr. and Mrs. D, not of them now, but as they appeared shortly after the birth of their last son, Randell. I could see proud parents and sleeping baby. Big plans, high expectations, good schools, tennis lessons, piano recitals, all the things attentive parents pour into their last best child, their baby.

And now where were they? I sat down at the desk and put Randell's chart in front of me. "Seventeen-year-old male, previously healthy, now with — " I stopped and tapped my pen against the paper. Now with what? Psychosis? Illusions? Hallucinations about the sewer system? A whole new and senseless world. I thought about Mr. and Mrs. D, who had unwittingly blundered into this other world, one they knew nothing about. This was a world of institutions, major tranquilizers, locked wards, disembodied voices.

For a moment I hated my job. Why do I have to be the one who breaks the news to these parents — that they may as well throw the Tough Love book out the window? That Randell's problems were an order of magnitude greater. Besides, maybe I'm wrong; I certainly am not a psychiatrist. But, still, I couldn't get out of my mind another alternate image of Mr. and Mrs. D, a dream almost. I could see them sitting in a dayroom somewhere in some psychiatric ward of some prestigious institution. They are there to visit their son and they are dressed up for this special occasion. They are nervous. They sit shoulder to shoulder and after a while the room starts to fill with patients, people whose paths the D's never dreamed they would cross: street people, the homeless, the psychotic, the depressed, muttering old women and stiff-gaited young men, the manic addicts, the zombies. The D's are sitting in this place, waiting for their son, holding each other's hands. It is here that they finally see that even if they gave their son all the love in the world, it still may not be enough.

ANGOR ANIMI

BY *John Stone, M.D.*

How long have I known this man, I thought, my head bowed, the crying over, done with, here in the hospital room; how long have I known this patient, this boy; this 22-year-old stretched out and quietly not breathing in the dark room. Raining outside. Seventeen years.

I first met David when he was five. I was then a Cardiology Fellow, learning how the heart works, how it goes wrong. I became his doctor some 10 years ago and over that time I came to think of him as something of a heroic figure. He'd been through three major orthopedic operations, two of them on his spine. And four years ago, the open-heart surgery that had allowed him to go back to school, to study microchips, computers, and other paraphernalia I know less and less about. He got on well after the surgery: quaffed a few on Saturday nights, went camping, went to the mountains. The trip he recalled with the greatest pleasure was one to the Gulf coast: he never forgot those five days with a college buddy, spent fishing, crabbing, cooking and eating. He liked the slower pace of that small town and told me later it was the kind of place he'd want to settle down in: the people there really knew how to live. I knew his heart wasn't perfect, never would be perfect. But there is, within the nation of Cardiology, the state of Perfect Enough: whatever works.

A month ago, almost matter-of-factly, after my office examination, he said that he was just a bit more short of breath. Not much, just a bit. A bit tired after climbing a flight of stairs. Still sleeping flat. Comfortable at rest. Maybe he was just putting on too much weight. Over the next few weeks, though, he got worse. He saw his family doctor with symptoms that sounded like flu, bronchitis. He seemed at first to respond to antibiotics. Cough got better. But then heart failure bore in on him. Air hunger. Having to sit up to catch his breath. And so he called me, or his mother called, and I admitted him to the hospital.

In the same hospital, four years before, he lay after his open-heart surgery, with pain at every breath because of the knife, his new heart valve working well. Post-op and sick. Breathing hard. But finally, as his mother and I watched, he began to come round. A little better every day. Tubes all out. Fever coming down without antibiotics. Stronger. Wanted a hamburger, a good sign, maybe the best sign. He strolled with me in the hall, nodding to the nurses, smiling gamely, talking about Dungeons and Dragons. He went back to school and did well: made the Dean's List one quarter and was very proud.

But now heart failure had descended on him like the plague. He had to work hard to breathe. In the Emergency Department, one of the Residents met me and helped me get an IV line in. The Resident was a physician I'd taken care of, several years ago, when he himself was sick and had to be hospitalized. I told David that the Resident never could get used to needles; he'd rebelled against needles, against my ordering too many blood tests. That seemed to reassure David, who only grimaced as the needle slipped into his own vein.

*   *   *

Over the next few days he improved. The treatment seemed to be working. He lost several pounds of fluid, began breathing easier. Sleeping flat. But almost as suddenly as it left, his difficulty came back. Tore into him with force. With recruitments. And he had to sit up again in order to breathe. Struggling for air. We got a scan of his heart and the confirmatory bad news. His heart was much bigger than it should be, barely pumping on the scan, pumping perhaps a third of what it should. Just enough to keep him alive.

I told his mother. Indirectly, I told David. Yes, the scan did show serious disease. Yes, I thought there were some things we could do to help him. No, we weren't licked yet. But I was afraid we were.

Morphine: a godsend. It works wonders. It does good things for the heart and the head. Though only temporarily, it brings respite from the heart failure. Slows the work of breathing, unloads the heart. It takes away the sensation of shortness of breath caused by fluid building up in the lungs, eases for a couple of hours or more the feeling of suffocation. Morphine works quickly and its actions are blessed: if you are still short of breath, you no longer care. You sleep. You dream.

On morning rounds today, David told me he'd seen some strange things outside his room in the middle of the night. He said he knew they weren't there. I asked him what kinds of things he saw. Dogs, he said; dogs and cats and a clown. I knew they weren't there, he said, because this is a hospital. Was it frightening? I asked. No, not frightening; it was kind of interesting. He'd been in the bustling beeping ICU too many days. But at least he'd recognized these hallucinations for what they were — or were not. We talked for a long time. He said he thought the new medicine was helping a bit. And the morphine really helps me, he said. Yes.

Angor Animi

71

✳   ✳   ✳

On my way out of the ICU, his mother called me into the waiting room. I told her about the dogs and cats and the clown. I told her I was worried. She was worn out from several straight nights spent between the waiting room and the ICU, smoothing back his sweaty hair, pouring soft drinks for him. Just being there. She'd told him that she had to go home for a while. Had to. Had to get a bath. Stretch out in bed for a few hours so that she could come back and continue to be with him. I agreed with her. She was red-eyed, exhausted. He didn't want her to leave him, of course. They'd argued briefly about that. She said to me, do you think he knows he's dying? Yes. Yes, I said. He knows; without being told. I wrote two Latin words on a 3 × 5 card for her: *angor animi* — Suetonius' phrase. It means the fear of impending doom, anguish of the spirit. Patients know. Yes, I said, he knows. But she did need to go home. She was no good here: to him or to herself. I sent her off.

At three o'clock, the office phone rang. It was the ICU nurse. David was worse; his blood pressure had fallen. Did I have any suggestions. I'll come, I said, slipping out the office door and walking briskly through the rain the one block to the hospital. Off the elevator and into the ICU. Oh, doctor; good, he said, as I came in. What's the matter, David? He was taking off the oxygen mask. Keep that on, David, you need it. He lay back on the bed, exhausted, sweating, his chest racked with the effort of breathing, the incredible energy of staying alive. As he lay down, his eyes rolled back just a bit too far in his head. I knew I had to call his mother. I went to the phone and dialed her quickly. She was on her way. I strode back into his room just as one of the nurses was coming out to get me, her face anxious. David had slumped further down and was taking a last quiet attempt at a breath. There was some initial flurry of activity around the bed, some confusion; the bag-valve-mask was put over his face and he was given some oxygen. But he was gone. No question. No more breaths on his own. I put my stethoscope on his chest. No movement of the chest. His EKG monitor was still going, but no breaths. I put the stethoscope back in my pocket, crossed my forearms on the bed rail, and the tears began welling up. I turned toward the window; raining outside. The staff had known what to expect; we'd talked at length: no heroics. No attempts at resuscitation. Let him go. Gracefully. Quietly. Which he had done. The tears came, the muffled noise in the throat, the sobs and gulpings, for several minutes. When I opened my eyes again, the staff had left the room, turning out the lights as they left. David lay peacefully. Like the *Pietà*, I thought, but waiting for his mother. I closed his eyes. We both waited.

One of the nurses who'd known David well, who'd cared for him for days and days, came into the room. We talked for a few minutes about his death, what needed to be done: details. Then, at the same time, we were both aware of an incongruity: the cardiac monitor, the EKG, was still showing some electrical activity. The cardiac impulses were still marching along across the screen in their electrical sweep. Should I turn off the monitor? she asked. Yes, I said, automatically. Yes. *No. No, wait. Turn it back on.* The EKG started its sweep across again. *Leave it on. His mother's on her way.* A minute later she came into the room. She already knew. *Angor animi.* She knew. Expected. Oh, David, my precious David, she said, gathering him to her, cradling him. Those are his last few beats, Judy, I said, pointing to the monitor. Just at that moment, as she looked, his heart stopped completely. He waited for you. She nodded, as though she'd expected that also. And perhaps she had. But I hadn't.

SOUTH BRONX
PEDIATRICS

BY *Susan Mates, M.D.*

Smells. You couldn't understand it without the smells. Car exhaust, rancid frying oil, fish, plantain. Urine, especially in the halls and corners. A splash of cheap perfume, alcohol breath so strong you might pass out. Vomit. Cigarette smoke. And still, with the only greening weeds punching up between sidewalk cracks and the pitiful malformed little trees along the curb, the dizzy smell of spring, fresh and warm, seeped through the dusted windows of the emergency room, cracked open as far as they could, with their arthritic eighty years, before they stuck. Smells accounted for a lot in the South Bronx.

He was a skinny, little Filipino doctor, Caraballo, about thirty-five, and we really hadn't even met. He kept to his small surgery, and I kept to my three pediatric examining rooms next door, which was a joke, since I had trained in Adult Medicine and got stuck in this dismal internship only because I ran out of money and had to graduate quick, almost a year before my real internship. Someone quit on them and it was the only job I could get. So, since the Filipino and I were alone in the peeling linoleum cubicles they called an emergency room, and since I had no idea what I was doing, occasional consultation was necessary.

Our little working area was across the Grand Concourse from

the big emergency room of City Hospital, where all the ambulances went, so we got only what could walk or be carried. Once I got a kid the cops had thrown out of the City emergency room for slugging the doctor, and his mother walked him across the street and was crying and begging me to see him — which, as you can imagine, I was none too pleased about. But there were legal issues, and, besides, there was her face, flushing and paling, her brown eyes commanding me. What kind of doctor is this little girl? I could see her thinking. She'd stopped with the boy in front of Caraballo on her way in. He was stitching up a drunk, and, short as he was, at least he was a man, and she was hoping to get him. Still, when she saw she had no choice, she focused on me with disgust and pleading.

For a half hour I stood and listened to the mother talk — how the boy has changed, how he's nervous all the time now, look at what just happened over at City, he's not that kind of boy. She was a short, sturdy woman from Puerto Rico, and she stood right in front of me, her legs planted apart, her voice rising every time I glanced out the door to the growing line of waiting kids. Croup, asthma, constipation, rashes. Two-day-old infants, five-year-olds, girls with trouble with their periods who would scream and faint when I told them they were pregnant. All the time the boy, who was a big, solid kid, was jumping and twitching and staring wild-eyed at me. Finally, I got the mother to leave the room and I looked directly at the kid, eyeball to eyeball, and said, "Okay, let's get this over with. Speed? Cocaine? Glue? Angel dust?"

"Nothing," he said, and I got a slightly uncomfortable feeling, nothing I could pin down. There it was again, the smells. Beer, urine, weed, a gentle April breeze with burned oil sifted through the window. I'd been wondering the whole time whether this kid was going to punch me, too. Our security was one old guard around the corner, not a real cop right in the room with you like at City.

"Really," the boy said to me, like he was going to cry. I looked up at him, trying to figure out why he wasn't cursing or spitting at me, or making any of the usual responses. That's when I saw it. I can still remember the way my heart stopped, my face heated up, the sweat dripped down my sides almost before what it was I was looking at hit my brain. The kid's thyroid was as big as a brick bulging out of his neck. His eyes were popping out from the disease, too. His blood pressure was probably through the roof. Jesus Christ. I'd been leisurely chatting up a boy in acute thyroid storm.

Right about this time the Filipino finished his stitching, peeled off his gloves, and strolled over to the half-open door of the examining room where we were. "Thyroid," he said. He'd already brought in the alcohol and four-by-fours and large-bore intravenous. He didn't say anything else, just helped me call the chief resident and the endocrine service, and talked to the mother in a soothing voice, although she actually looked quite relieved now that we were as excited as she was. Finally, we shipped the boy upstairs.

"It took me a half hour, and it was right in my face," I said, shaking now that I knew the kid would be okay. Caraballo, who'd done a rotating internship in Manila, plus who knows how many years of what kind of practice, just shrugged his shoulders. We were the same height, but he was wiry and I outweighed him by at least twenty pounds. He looked tired and went back to his room. You could be the best doctor in the whole Philippines, but if you came to America, you took a test ten times harder than the one the Americans took, and you got to start all over, in the worst internships, the ones Americans wouldn't even touch.

As it happened, one of my friends was on duty at City that night, so later on I called her up and said, "Guess what you guys missed, ha ha ha. His thyroid was so big it looked like a spare tire around his neck, and his eyes were bulging right out of the sockets." I didn't mention the half-hour chat at all.

After that, I began to pay more attention to Caraballo. He looked lonely to me, and oppressed. I smiled at him when we passed in the hall, and asked him his opinion of cases with graciousness and formality, to show that I knew, even if the rest of the ignorant staff did not, that a short man, even a Filipino, could be a good doctor. I felt a solidarity with him, me, a woman in those days when there were so few, and him, another undesirable. I thought perhaps he had a crush on me.

It was a horrible time. I was terrified going to work. I had been promised a supervising resident when I took the job because I had told the director the truth, which is that I knew no pediatrics. Instead, they put me, alone, except for the surgeon, in the emergency room. The nurse was a big Irish woman, about fifty, with spidery red veins across her cheeks, and white hair. She must have had some sympathy for me, because she would write nursing assessments like "croupy cough, needs mist tent," when I had no idea how to diagnose croup, or "chicken pox, contagious" or "strep throat, penicillin." Most of the parents knew what the kids had better than I did. The nurse would feed me English biscuits with butter on them, and whisper what to do. She didn't like the Filipino.

Once, a man who was a phlebotomist for a living at one of the big private hospitals brought in his eight-year-old girl seizing. He was pretty agitated even when he got there, but we gathered that he had stopped giving her her seizure medicine just out of sheer laziness. He was Haitian, and big. The nurse and I got the girl flat on a table, and I tried to get a vein. Her arms were flailing, and I was not too good at starting IVs in kids yet, although I wasn't too bad either. It was a feeling of extreme torture, trying to hit a moving target while calculating how many milligrams per kilogram of Valium to give. I've never been good at doing arithmetic in my head, let alone when the answer is life or death and I'm trying to get a tiny vein in a jerking arm with a needle.

I'd stuck her a few times when the father decided to go berserk. "I can do better than that," he yelled at me. "You don't know what you're doing. You're not a real doctor."

I was still trying to hold down the girl, calculate the dose, watch her breathing, and get that IV slid into place. He grabbed my arm and pulled me away. I was trying to control myself, to focus on this girl, to do this thing, to get through it, and, dear God, not let her die. The nurse grabbed the father and clawed at him. "Get out of the room," she shouted. "What do you think you are doing touching the doctor?"

The girl was turning a little blue around the lips now, her neat braids fuzzy from jerking against the litter. She had surprisingly clear and lovely skin, radiant, like a ripe plum. Her eyes were rolled back and saliva strung out from the corner of her mouth. Even as I got the butterfly needle in, taped it, pushed the Jesus-I-hoped-it-was-the-right-dose-of Valium in, her father got me around the throat and pulled me back. The nurse lunged for the intravenous, to keep it in, and it held, and the girl jerked a few more times and stopped. The father was choking me with his huge arm, and I was tearing at him and still watching the girl: Was she going to stop breathing? Maybe I didn't get the dose right. We had to do the intubations ourselves those days, and the tiny pediatric tubes were taped against the wall like talismans. I'd looked at them every night and looked away. I'd done two or three adult intubations, but never a child.

Suddenly the father let me go. Without even looking back, I staggered over to the girl, who was sleeping now. I checked her breathing, her pulse, her blood pressure, her color. She was okay. I told the nurse to call the resident and bring her upstairs, and I brushed past the father and ran to the bathroom, down the hall, where the line of people in the waiting room couldn't see me. I threw up.

When I came back, the father tried to apologize but I told him to get out. "You should have given her her medicine," I shouted. "Leave." Then I called up the director of the program. "I should have a pediatric resident backing me up," I shouted. "It's not right. This is no way to run an emergency room. It's immoral. I won't do it anymore."

"Watch your tongue, young woman," the director said. "You can be replaced."

When I hung up the phone, Caraballo was looking at me through the doorway to his surgery. "Should, should, should," he said, after a minute. "You want to talk about should, maybe you should memorize the doses of important medicines."

I was on a roll now. A few weeks later, the chief resident refused to admit a boy with asthma and pneumonia, even though there was an open bed. She didn't want to inconvenience the admitting resident, who was a friend of hers. They were both from Argentina, and made rounds in Spanish. I smiled and, as soon as she left, called the chief resident of every other hospital in the Bronx until one of them admitted the boy, over census, to the hallway. The next day their director complained to ours. That afternoon, our chief resident changed the on-call schedule. I was now on call twice as often as any other intern, and on every holiday within striking distance.

"Boy, that's not right," I said to Caraballo. "I'm going to quit." But I didn't, because I had no other job and I was still dead broke. The Filipino listened to my shouting, shrugged his shoulders, and told me he was on all the time, with no time off. He was the only surgeon for the emergency room, and lived in the hospital, except holidays, when they got a moonlighter to cover him.

As the year went on, I visited Caraballo more. Sometimes, when I got some sleep, I would bake cookies and bring them in for us to share, or I would go over and watch him work, with his meticulous fingers, suturing, examining, touching. He wasn't much of a talker, although I gathered that in his opinion Manila emergency rooms were much worse than anything in the South Bronx. I figured he had to be pretty lonely, in a foreign country, no family, working so hard. I talked a lot about how the administration ran the hospital, poor people, capitalism, and right and wrong. He ate the cookies.

It was when we had gained this rapport, or so I thought, that the gun incident occurred. Afterward, the staff said they could feel it coming, the weather had gone so suddenly from breezy spring to hot, humid summer. We were in the fifth day of a heat wave and it was only June. The air sat thick and heavy, so still it didn't matter whether the windows were opened or closed, except for the noise. Closed, you sweated with every move and heard the murmur of the waiting room, the groans of patients in surgery, the crying babies, and the page system of the hospital. Open, you sweated with every move, heard all that, and also the horns, the sirens, and the thump of salsa music from the bar across the street.

Smells intensified in the humidity, body odors of urine and sweat and bad breath. Street smells of steamy pavement, of meals cooked that morning, last night, decades ago — tomato sauces, boiled cabbage, sausage, tortilla, tongue, frying oil. Spanish, Irish, Polish, Jewish, smells going back to farmlands and horse manure, the quiet, sweet smell of the land when you could still taste the sea across the South Bronx. Our security guard sat, peeled down to his undershirt, with the men from housekeeping out on the front steps of the hospital. The neighborhood was on the street, housewives with thin white blouses stuck to their backs dragging shopping carts and red-faced children, whores leaning, sweating against the blackened buildings, dealers and pimps gunning Cadillac convertibles, a pair of cops dripping in their blue uniforms, walking. And all in languorous motion, heavy and waiting.

Inside, it was slow, too hot to get sick, or to do anything about it. I'd drifted into Caraballo's surgery. I thought I'd make my big move, invite him across the street for lunch. The nurse rolled her eyes but told me to go ahead, she'd yell out the window if she needed us. We had beepers but they broke all the time, so shouting worked better. The Filipino was standing near the locked medicine cabinet checking the sterile packs. A week before, a bullet to the chest came in and Caraballo couldn't find a clean thoracotomy kit. He didn't say a lot about it, but after that he'd checked the stack of green, cloth-wrapped, autoclaved kits every day. I was standing closer to the door, making small talk and sweating in my white coat.

I first noticed something was wrong by Caraballo's sudden yank to attention. His eyes were fixed on the doorway. I turned to look, and that's when I saw the gun. It was small and gray. Strangely small, after all the movies and comic books and reports on the evening news. Afterward, I always thought of the first time a man exposed himself to me, and how long it took me to realize that the little, limp, pink thing he was flipping around was a penis. I suppose some men expose themselves erect, but none of them ever chose me. Anyway, here was a tall, gaunt young man pointing his tiny gun at us. It was C. J. Rodriguez. We got to know him later, and he wasn't so bad, just a doper needing his fix, and really kind of sweet and pathetic, but we didn't know that at the time. He was hunched over, like he had watched too many cop shows, and his nut-brown hands were shaking wildly as he aimed at Caraballo. For a long time, all I saw was the hole at the end of that gray barrel.

"Open it, fucker," C.J. croaked. There was sweat dripping down his face and just running off. He had a little pencil mustache and unshaven cheeks, but still he didn't look mean, just crazy.

That's when I noticed Caraballo. He was standing directly in front of the medicine cabinet with his arms crossed, staring at C.J. and shaking his head. "No," he said.

South Bronx Pediatrics

"What do you mean, 'no'?" I hissed, trying to ease my way toward the door, where the nurse was holding up a paper towel reading, "Security coming." Great, I thought. Between Caraballo and our old broken-down security guard we were definitely going to get shot. "Caraballo," I said, "just let him have the morphine."

"No," said Caraballo. He had a look of great calm on his face, as if this were the Zen of emergency room work.

C.J. was really shaking now, his nose was running, and he looked about ready to die. He kept pointing the gun at Caraballo. "Come on, man," he said, almost pleading, "open it up and I'm out of here."

"No," said the Filipino, standing perfectly still. Then all hell broke loose. The security guard, a huge, old Pole who used to be a meat packer, drew his own gun, ran at C.J., and tried to tackle him from behind. To this day I don't know why he did both, draw his gun and tackle, but it wasn't a good idea. The two of them went down and C.J.'s eyes widened as the shot came from the security guard's gun. C.J.'s arm hit the floor and his gun went off a second later, so it sounded almost like two parts of the same shot, "crack-crack," really close together. I closed my eyes from pain, the sound was so loud in the tiled operating room.

When I collected myself, it looked like a battlefield. Caraballo had been shot in the foot, C.J. in the thigh, and the security guard had broken his arm when he hit the floor. Our nurse was tut-tutting and picking up the guns like they were contaminated, while the upstairs surgical resident, an orthodox Jew named Ira, who was there because they let him have Saturdays off, ran to Caraballo and felt over his foot, then pressure-dressed it and paged the attending stat. All this time C.J. lay there curled up like a baby, whimpering and bleeding. It was Caraballo who finally grunted at Ira and pointed to C.J. Ira rolled his eyes and went over and started cutting off C.J.'s pant leg, looking for the wound.

It must have been twenty minutes later or so, and I was trying to hold the pressure on Caraballo's foot when a plump Filipino woman hurtled through the door, followed by two doll-like children dressed in lace. She said something to Caraballo in what I assumed was Tagalog. He answered, laughing, even though he looked about to faint. She said something briefly again, then pushed each little girl forward to kiss his clammy forehead and she herself bent over to kiss his cheek, and they left.

When the attending surgeon came running in, his shirt still unbuttoned, they sent C.J. upstairs, where another surgeon operated on him. Then C.J. stayed for a couple of months because it turned out he had nowhere to go. The Filipino, on the other hand, they did right in his own operating room, under local. The last thing I saw before they closed the door was our Irish nurse saying, "You have such darling children," to him, as if they were at a cocktail party, all the while washing the area around his foot with betadine and ignoring his groans. She'd been working in the ER a long time.

I got caught up on my patients, several of whom complained about the long wait even though they had a front-row view of the doctors getting shot up, and went back to the surgery just as Caraballo was being wheeled out by the surgical resident from upstairs. I caught Ira's hand and stopped him. The Filipino looked up at me.

"Why?" I said.

Caraballo looked pale but he smiled a sharp-toothed smile at that. "Because," he said, "it was the *right* thing to do."

"It was stupid," I shouted after him, but they had already gone out the front door to where I presume his wife was waiting with the car.

I finally did quit the next day and got a job waiting tables at the Italian restaurant up the street until my real internship started the next year. The one that counted, the one in medicine. Sometimes, on my CV, I round time periods off to years, so that the South Bronx Pediatrics just disappears, and it looks like I went straight from medical school to a reputable program in medicine. It's easier that way, not to have to explain.

TEACHING ROUNDS

BY *Lawrence Schneiderman, M.D.*

This morning on rounds I learn that a patient has died because of a mistake made by the ward team during the night. They are visibly upset when they tell me this. I am sad about the patient, of course, a young man with AIDS, but I am even more concerned about the impact of this mistake on the doctors I am teaching, young residents and their acolyte students. The patient was about to die in any case, whereas my trainees have their whole professional life ahead of them. Medicine is a terrible taskmaster, imposing an unrealistic standard of perfection. I try to soften the blow by telling them, "If it's true you learn from your mistakes, someday I will know everything."

I like the sound of my voice when I say this. It conveys a combination of dignity and humility, appropriate for an attending physician who wants to command respect and at the same time bridge the gap to the young. We sit in the doctor's office, surrounded by medical records, they in their scruffy, slept-in whites, I in my Brooks Brothers suit. Their eyes are wide with appreciation. These are teaching rounds. I regard them as a sacred time and, following a tradition I inherited from my own great teachers of the past, I instruct the ward clerk and nurses to interrupt us only for the most dire emergencies.

During these sessions I often make use of stories from my own life as a doctor-in-training. Once dismissed as mere anecdotes, such stories are now called narratives and are highly regarded in academic centers as important teaching techniques. Today, I draw from my file of stories: Mistakes I Made Back When I Was in Your Shoes. A woman with cancer who died a terrible death from intestinal obstruction because I neglected to pay attention to her bowels while treating her pain with large doses of morphine. A young woman with urinary tract infection who died suddenly of gram negative sepsis while I dithered over which antibiotic to give her. I learned from these mistakes, I tell them. Now I know better. Always check the bowels when you're giving morphine, and never dither when there's a possibility of gram negative sepsis. This morning I tell them about another young man, Ramon Romita.

I was an intern when I first saw Ramon one Sunday morning in Emergency. For some reason he could not get over the flu. Tough, cocky, captain of his high school basketball team, Ramon planned to make use of the summer to perfect his skills while working for Parks and Recreation. He was hoping, his family was hoping, everyone in his high school was hoping he would come back senior year and lead his team to a championship. But early in July he began to have trouble keeping up with his buddies. He had lost his speed, his moves, his strength, his endurance. When he lost his jump shot he agreed to see a doctor.

The neighborhood doctor he consulted gave him a shot of penicillin and sent him on his way. When that didn't work the doctor went through his cabinet of free samples to no avail. By the time I saw him a week or so later in Emergency he could barely climb onto the examining table. I was less than a month into my training, but after noting his fever and rapid pulse on his ER sheet and observing his pasty, bloodless flesh, his shambling struggles, and after feeling the lump of spleen, I already had a good idea of what was going on. His mother and father followed every move I made with frightened scowls. Something was terribly wrong, and they were right. Their son had acute leukemia.

Right away I played God. For starters I used the word "leukemia" without collapsing. They, being mere mortals, surely would have collapsed if I had not already sat them down. Then, in a voice I knew was as awesome as it was calm, I explained to them what was happening, why Ramon was weak and tired (his oxygen-carrying red cells had dropped to about a third of normal), why he had fever (there were so many leukemic white cells they were heating his body up like a crowded bus). I answered their flailing questions with precise words that staked down their wind-blown fears. I spoke of miracles. We had drugs, powerful drugs that could fight off the disease, chase it away. Right there in front of them I put in a page for Hematology-Oncology. I told the Romitas I would see to everything.

From that day forth the whole family locked in on me as their miracle worker. *El Salvador.* And even though Ramon's chemotherapy was being directed by Heme-Onc, the family agreed to nothing, no change in medications, no alteration of dose, no blood test, no X ray, without first checking with me. We had bonded, as the fashionable phrase goes. All the other doctors and nurses knew this and accepted it — happily, for it freed them from the tedium of donning sterile cap, gown, mask, and gloves every time a blood culture had to be drawn or a festering rectum probed or a transfusion line unplugged. Most of all it freed them from having to answer the hundreds of daily questions and complaints.

Even though I was only an intern amid battalions of celebrated specialists, no less than *el Salvador* was I, the one who first reached out his hand, touched their son's wilting body, spoke the words and raised him. *El Salvador.* Even though the terrible stuff I caused to be dripped into his veins made him sick as hell for weeks. For it seemed not only to serve as further proof of my powers, but also to satisfy a deep sense of Manichean drama, that the purging of evil required such dreadful cataclysms.

But Ramon, as it turned out, was on the wrong side of the percentages. He had the most ruthless form of leukemia. And although I always couched my daily reports in what I thought was realistic optimism, I was no fool: It was the optimism everyone heard, not the realism. We were all joined in an unspoken conspiracy against fate. Didn't I tell them miracles were possible? Ramon was going to beat the odds, now, during basketball season, and ever after.

And Ramon did get better. He even returned to Parks and Recreation before the summer was over and resumed playing basketball. No one expected him right away to be as sharp as he was before he got sick, so every successful jump shot, every stolen pass, every rebound that fell into his hands served as a confirming sign from heaven. Rare, yes, but how often do *you* receive signs from heaven?

The first relapse occurred just after school had started. Because we were following his blood counts closely we could tell when things were going sour even before Ramon could. Despite the minor rebellion in the outlying provinces of the blood, he, Ramon, safe in the central capital, was getting stronger, taller, handsomer every day. A sheen of black hair, a downy hint of Don Juan mustache. His parents could not contain their gratitude, and the aunts and uncles and sisters and cousins who surrounded him in their shimmery dresses and shirts and plied me with Mexican pastries were like celebrants at Lourdes or Fatima.

And once again the magic worked. We treated the relapse with another batch of witches' brew, and within a month I could tell the Romitas that the leukemic white cells had been chased away. If the Romitas were believers before, now they were idolaters. My sessions with the Romita faithful could have been painted on the ceiling of the Sistine Chapel.

Did I actually believe this nonsense myself? I'm afraid I did. I was trapped in it as much as they were. I had already become this young basketball star. Were not the two of us — prancy and snazzy as we were — put on earth to live? Old geezers in other rooms were finishing their tour, but surely not young studs like us. It made no sense. Especially when every week or so another bestseller came out declaring that all you had to do was *think positively,* make those silly little cancer cells laugh and roll helplessly on the floor while you *took charge of your life!* Maybe — no, not maybe — *yes,* there would be a miracle, *yes* he would survive. *Yes,* I would be forgiven for allowing this bloated reverence for life and this obscene reverence for me to go unchecked.

Then came the final relapse, the most terrible day of reckoning. Ramon showed up again in Emergency, looking worse than ever, more pasty and shambling, his hair sopping wet with fever, his heart thrashing almost audibly in the room, his spleen this time so engorged it could be seen bulging out of his belly. I arranged to have him admitted.

The Romitas all chipped in to pay for a private room and packed it with a fiesta-day crowd — faces shiny with expectation, primped for the occasion in holiday suits and colorful dresses — awaiting the arrival of *el Salvador* and his next miracle. They landscaped the room with sweet-smelling flowers and dazzling paper imitations. They brought in extra chairs, crowded along the windowsill, pressed around his bed, squeezed his hands, rubbed his feet. When I arrived, all sound ceased, a path parted for me, and I entered bearing my talismans, an IV tray and two units of blood.

And there, before the throng of worshipers, I failed. By then, my reputation for locating a delicate vein amid Ramon's fibrous tangles had become legendary. *El Salvador,* unlike those clumsy lab techs, gave one swift stroke and was in, followed customarily by a chorus of sighs and Ramon's assertion that he didn't feel a thing. A small deed, true, but one of heroic proportions to ordinary mortals who faint at scratches.

But this time my suave thrust came up dry. I prodded about with my finger. The needle seemed to be in the right place. But it was unaccountably insubordinate. Perhaps a minute plane of tissue separated it from the vein. I pushed, causing a small outcry. I wiggled, tugged at the skin, nothing. Nothing except pain, and more pain, which made me cringe along with Ramon, as though the needle were clawing inside *me*. Meanwhile I could feel my fingers grow cold and lose their safecracker's touch. I became aware of a silence consolidating behind my back, a dreadful silence, a dark doom that mocked the Romitas' festive preparations. (Would they ever again wear those shimmery shirts and dresses, those flowery ties, without remembering?) For the first time they saw the battle turning against them, their god sprawled before the gods of their enemy.

Again and again I failed — meanwhile never willing to admit defeat, never calling for help — while Ramon, who finally could take it no longer, unleashed an endless torrent of curses. The Romitas saw their god abject and helpless. And so I was. With me still yanking the needle back and forth under Ramon's howls, he died, cringing and squirming. To my shame, it never occurred to me, *el Salvador,* to show mercy, give him morphine and let him stretch out and pass away in peace.

"And so you see," I tell my ward team, shaking my head ruefully, bringing my cautionary tale to its conclusion, "the most lasting lessons come from our mistakes. Ramon taught me the lesson of pride. If it's true you learn from your mistakes, someday I'll know everything."

I have told that story many times to many doctors-in-training. But this time as I look around the silent room I note something odd in those wide eyes, eyes that I thought had been gazing at me appreciatively. Is there a glint of ironic amusement? Even something harder — a bloodshot, weary anger? They know I do not like it when they are sloppy (I myself always make a point of wearing only a new or freshly pressed suit), yet there they are, slouching almost defiantly in their slept-in hospital uniforms. What are they thinking? I wonder. And I hear my stately voice still hanging in the air. *The lesson of pride.* The lesson of pride, indeed.

And I think, Some lessons are so hard to learn. And I see the struggling Ramon striving to teach me still.

CELEBRITY MEDICINE

BY *Ethan Canin, M.D.*

I was working in the emergency room on an overnight shift when the surgeon on duty pointed to a room where the curtain had been drawn closed and told me that an interesting man had just come in: "I'd like your opinion," he said.

This was in 1988 at the Brigham and Women's Hospital in Boston, a labyrinth of a place, which, because it was a sophisticated university center on the edge of a poor neighborhood, tended to a vast range of people. The emergency room saw winos and shooters and the down-and-out, just like any emergency room in that kind of neighborhood, but because it was a teaching hospital it also saw a fair number of patients who came in the back door with private bodyguards. We were always hearing of princes and presidents and movie stars being brought in, and more than once I was asked to leave an elevator by security men. I was just a fourth-year medical student at the time, and in the emergency room I spent most of my shifts sewing up cuts. People didn't ever ask me my opinion unless they wanted to point out my ignorance.

"I'd like to know what you think," said the surgeon, a buoyant, mischievous man who liked to ask for my assistance on the really bloody cases, men who'd been hit by trucks or caught in boat blades, just to see if I could stand it. "He's quite a man."

"Where's the chart?"

"He doesn't have a chart."

"Everybody has a chart."

He winked at me. "This is an unusual man."

I was in scrubs, smelly from my all-night shift, my pockets stuffed with latex gloves and suture packages for the cuts I saw, but when I knocked and went in I found a wealthy-looking man in a fine suit, pacing along the wall. He looked to be in his sixties, and he had on an ascot and a fedora. I couldn't see anything wrong with him.

"Boy, am I glad to see you," he said. "I've just gotten off the plane — remind me to tell you about that. It's not something I should tell you but I might anyway." He pulled out a leather briefcase that was under the bed and tapped it. "It's why I can't let this out of my sight."

"What brings you to the hospital, sir?"

He looked closely at me. "I can tell you're a trustworthy man," he said.

I tucked in my scrub shirt. "Thank you."

"We were going over the numbers. We were all there, except the one everybody wants to know about. He hardly ever comes along, but O'Neill and Rebozo and Darman were there. Notice those names — Democrats and Republicans together. That's why he can't be seen there. That's why we meet on the plane. I'm their egghead economist. Have you ever heard of me?"

"No, sir."

"Of course not. That's how I like to keep it. But you've heard of Rebozo." He clapped his hands together. "That's because he *wants* you to know about him. He's the fly in the cheese. He can't keep it quiet. The way to get things done is to stay out of the way in those types of things. I tell Darman what my projections are and he takes credit for them. That doesn't bother me. I could care less. What's more important is the budget, not my personal fame. That's how you make a budget when everybody wants a different thing, O'Neill and Bradley and Dole. Rebozo doesn't understand that. That's why the thing almost didn't work. And that's why you've heard of him and not me."

I was trying my new technique of trying to figure out what was wrong with a patient by having a normal conversation. I'd been taught that a good doctor could discern a fair number of diagnoses just by chatting — neurological problems, heart and lung problems, endocrine problems — but this gentleman seemed vigorous and educated and, well, healthy. He looked a good deal less sick than I suspected *I* did.

"What were you deciding about the budget?" I asked.

He took off his hat and held it upside down in his palm, like a polite cowboy, then put it back on his head. He lowered his voice. "The glue that's tripping the horses is capital gains," he whispered. "Moynihan wants twenty-eight percent and five years and O'Neill wants thirty-two without the phaseout and Darman says three years and Helms says none. I'm the lineman. I push a hole through that wall." He opened his briefcase, shielding it from me, then closed it again.

"So what brings you to the hospital tonight?" I said again.

He smiled. "I think Moynihan will come south and Helms will come north, which makes Darman look like the one. That's my prediction. Take that to the stock market if you invest. Do you?"

"Do I invest? No, sir."

"Good, you're too smart for that. But a word to the wise — if the boys think inflation's beat, you help the cyclicals."

"Thank you."

He stepped up close. "I'd like to pay you for your help."

"That's all right, sir."

"No, it's not. They pay you nothing for this. I know." He took off the fedora again and this time pulled out a roll of bills from the crown. They were bent an inch thick around a gold clip, and as he leaned forward I saw that they were hundreds. He pulled off the first one and held it out. "Please."

"I couldn't, sir," I said, but even as I spoke I wondered if this was true. My income was nowhere near what I paid for rent and tuition.

"Of course you can." He plucked up another hundred in his fingers and began to separate it from the roll. "No," he said suddenly, stepping back. "That would be unethical. You're too honest for that." He looked down at his briefcase. "Would you be kind enough to leave me alone for a moment?"

"I'll be right back, sir."

Outside, I looked again for his chart but he really didn't seem to have one. I wandered out into the hallway outside the emergency room, debating about the money and wondering how I would describe him to the surgeon in charge. The truth was, I realized, I still hadn't discovered what was wrong with him. I'd already spent too much time in there and didn't want to go back in to find out an answer to the most basic question: Why was he here?

When I came back into the emergency room I said to the surgeon, "He's interesting, all right. He's one of the President's economic advisers. He's quite a wealthy man himself. I'm not sure I should have been the one to see him."

He smiled at me, raising his eyebrows. "What else?"

I raised my own. "He tried to pay me."

"I was wondering whether you'd tell me that." He held up a chart that he'd had in his hand. "He always tries to pay me too. Did you take it?"

"No."

"He does it every time he comes in. He has a roll of bills as thick as your wrist."

"Hundreds," I said. "Two inches thick. It must be ten thousand dollars. He comes in a lot?"

He opened the chart. "He comes in three or four times a year," he said, "always around the first of the month." He closed the chart again. "Now why would that be?"

I tried to think of a disease that would be related to the first of the month. "I don't know."

"Think about it. Why would he choose that day?"

I thought of endocrine cycles, menstrual cycles, and what psychiatrists call anniversary reactions. "I don't know," I said again.

"Because that's when the Social Security checks go out," he said. He sat down and opened the chart for me. "He's a manic-depressive," he explained. "He's off his lithium on a mania and making this all up."

"He's quite a liar then."

"Most of them are. It's one of the signs."

"And he's still a rich man."

"Hardly. He gets five hundred thirty dollars a month. That's standard SSI. Then he cashes the check into four hundreds and a hundred-and-thirty ones. There are just four hundred-dollar bills on the top of the roll. The rest are ones."

I looked down. It was a moment of learning.

"Welcome to the world of mania," said the surgeon. "The poor guy lives in a residence hotel with a bare lightbulb on the ceiling and a drawer full of lithium. The rest is just his mind."

I looked over at the cubicle, where now he was peeking out the curtain at us. I'd had the feeling in there of being around an extraordinary man, the kind of man who actually could be deciding the fate of a country, flying around with senators, and I believe it changed my view of the world that day to understand his fancy suddenly as a quirk of brain chemistry. It was the first time I'd ever seen a manic-depressive in the midst of a mania, the first time I'd ever seen the imploring charm and astounding inventiveness of the unfettered imagination. He truly could have been who he said, as far as I was concerned, so fluent was his knowledge and so captivating his energy, but now through the window I could see that he knew we were talking about him. He touched his ascot and stepped back from view. My job would be to call the psychiatrist and get him started again on his lithium. In those days I wasn't yet used to an emergency room. It was a small thing but it broke my heart.

THE HUNT

BY *Manjula Jeyapalan, M.D.*

Trauma one! Trauma one! En route five minutes," a voice from my pager boomed. Sounds of panic awakened me from a deep sleep. I had placed the pager on the bare windowsill, hoping that it would not summon me to another night on call, another night without sleep, another gunshot victim. Outside it was dark and melancholy. Through the open window, I saw a few lights in an adjacent building twinkling like stars in a dark sky. I stumbled from the bed, feet groping for the shoes. Slipping them on, I made my way into the hallway and rushed toward the emergency room. Others had been alerted as well — nurses, residents, and technicians, racing, like myself, toward the trauma room. I wanted to be the winner in this race for high stakes — against time, against death. I was first at the supply wall to don shoe covers. There was such a clamor of voices, such an articulation of commands and such a shouting of names. Goggle-eyed and double-gloved, I waited with fellow team members for the emergency medicine technicians to arrive.

So many trauma cases and practically overwhelming on a Friday night, when the hunters and the hunted, mostly young men of diverse ethnicities — Laotian, Hispanic, Black, White, and Cambodian — hang around the dark streets because they have nothing better to do. They are all hopeless youth who, at the slightest provocation, go at each other with their hands or whatever weapons they hold. Now and then it happens that the weapons are assault rifles. Then, the hunted don't have a chance. Who should it be this time? I wondered: old or young, rich or poor, girl or boy?

The entrance door swung open and three EMTs burst through it, wheeling a boy on a gurney. He was rigged to an intravenous tube cascading down from a pole alongside. One of the three shouted, "Thirteen-year-old Hispanic male, status post gunshot wound in the right flank; found conscious at the scene; vital signs stable . . ."

I stood there spellbound and saddened by the sight of the victim — so young a boy, so small for his age. He was screaming and writhing on the gurney.

"It's unfair," I said.

"What is?" responded a male voice to my involuntary remark.

"He being so young and already a victim," I replied.

"I've seen even younger victims," whispered the voice in the same cold and casual tone that profaned me. I felt an outrage that translated into a scowl.

Medical procedures started to swing into motion: Intravenous access was obtained, a rectal examination done, and a Foley placed. I picked up the admit sheet and began, in an unsteady hand, the history and physical. But more commotion and noise interrupted and another gurney swept through with another boy, slightly older. Snippets of their story were rearranged in my confused mind. The two were members of a gang. They had been sitting in a car on a Friday night awaiting fun, excitement, adventure, and romance. Instead, they became sitting ducks for the hunters. In a mood that mixed fury with sadness, I returned to the interrupted task of taking the first victim's history. I asked him if he hurt and he shouted, "All over . . . all over. . . . Do something to stop the pain!"

His name was Juan Carlos, a Mexican boy recently inducted

into a Laotian gang. His hair was closely cropped, in appearance like a Buddhist monk, but in behavior so different. There was a strange fearlessness in the pair of black eyes that glared at me.

"Another car pulled up and opened fire. We didn't do nothing," he sniveled.

"Did you have any weapons?" I asked.

"No!" he replied violently.

The policeman standing beside him said wryly, "We found him with a loaded gun in the backseat of the car."

Two X-ray technicians came in and we went behind screens to watch X rays being taken of Juan Carlos's abdomen and chest. The X rays concluded, the technicians left. A resident threw me a peritoneal lavage kit. A nasogastric tube and Foley had already been placed earlier. I put the boy in Reverse Trendelenberg, prepped and draped him, numbed the skin site and advanced the catheter. How many times had I done the same routine, over and over again? Even though I had been in the trauma unit for only a month, I could perform the procedures with my eyes closed. Of all the victims I had seen so far, Juan Carlos was the youngest. How could someone so young become the target of such hate? Whom did he hate and why? He would not stop moaning and groaning. The more I poked and probed, the more he hurt. I knew that it was annoying him. I explained to him that it was necessary to determine if there was blood in his abdomen. If there was, we needed to send him to the operating room to prevent further internal bleeding.

I hung the bag of saline and went to the box area to see his X rays. My chief, Dr. Harris, was already there reading them. In the center of the abdominal radiograph, there was a metallic-dense object lodged in the third lumbar vertebral body. Something was odd about the long bones. They had a funny lucent area at the distal ends. My first thought was that they were somehow diseased. Then it struck me that the epiphyseal ends had not yet fused because the boy had not reached puberty. Even the sight of the lead bullet and the circumstances in which he was shot could not erase the thoughts of his innocence from my mind. I returned to the trauma room. Juan Carlos was still groaning. The saline had almost emptied. I removed it from the rack and laid it on the ground next to the gurney. The bag began to refill slowly.

Suddenly, the door opened and a slightly built, shabby, and graying woman came in, dragging behind her a younger woman. So unkempt they were that both women had the appearance of having been pulled out of a trash bin. The older woman, his mother, in frantic grief and despair, ran up to Juan Carlos and stroked his hairless head while jabbering in Spanish. She tried to make herself pleasant and endearing to her boy, but Juan Carlos gave no sign of knowing, seeing, or hearing her. He stared at the ceiling without blinking his large eyes. She did not know how to communicate with her son and addressed me instead. An indefinable something in the scenario suggested that Juan Carlos came from a single-parent household. His male heroes and role models were outside his home. In broken English, she told me that he had dropped out of school last year and joined a gang and how hard she had tried to keep her son away from it.

"As a member of gang, he somebody; without gang, he says, he nobody."

Ignoring the pleas of this gentle and deferential woman, Juan Carlos had joined a gang. The younger woman, Juan Carlos's sister, interrupted. She could not conceal from me her true feelings about her brother. Between sobs, she said he was a terrible encumbrance to their mother, herself, and two other brothers, both much younger than Juan Carlos. She hoped they would not follow in his footsteps. I listened to her without comment or motion of body — a stillness induced by deep concern for this family's well-being. To assuage their sorrow, distress, pain, worries, fears, frustrations, helplessness, and despair, I told the sobbing women that

The Hunt

Juan Carlos was lucky. The bullet, on its ravaging course, had avoided vital organs and lodged itself in the vertebra. Juan Carlos stirred. His taut figure seemed to relax and, I thought, I saw a smile cross his face. He had survived the "hit" — the bullet fired by the enemy. That was an achievement in itself. He had shown himself to be invincible. He would be better liked by members of his gang and move up rapidly within it. He had the bullet in him to show and tell.

Juan Carlos's friend was not so lucky. We spent the rest of the night in the operating room trying to save his life. We removed most of his pancreas, his spleen, resected part of his bowel, and put a stitch in his liver.

Juan Carlos was placed on the pediatric floor and his friend in the Intensive Care Unit. I saw both every morning. I looked forward to the visits, especially to Juan Carlos. His cherublike face seemed to glow more as each day went by and he got better. I told Dr. Harris that I was happy he had survived with so little amiss. His cynical reply was, "Why? He'll go out there again and get killed."

"No, he won't. Once bitten, twice shy," I said.

"Oh, yeah!" he replied. "A gunshot wound is a distinguished fate for any member of a youth gang; it brings recognition and fame. He's bound to return to the scene of the crime, and those who missed the target the first time will fire, again and again, until they get it right."

Even in this mood of acute hopelessness, Dr. Harris audibly wondered what he could do to save Juan Carlos from his predatory friends.

"Think twice about whom you hang out with," he advised. "Your friend in the ICU is in great pain. He's lost his spleen, most of his pancreas, and is pooping into a bag dangling from his abdominal wall."

How harsh and cruel those words rang in my ears. Juan Carlos stared, with rage in his heart and the bullet in his vertebra. His large, staring eyes confronted Dr. Harris like two suns emitting relentless flames. Dr. Harris, without the slightest change in his sour disposition, walked out of the room and I followed him, deeply resentful of his callous attitude. Sensing my feelings, Dr. Harris told me that I should not let emotions interfere with my judgment.

"You stabilize, treat, and release them and hope to God they won't return."

A week had gone by since Juan Carlos was admitted to the ER. Now he seemed much better and was recuperating well. When we walked into his room in the morning, his behavior confirmed our favorable prognosis. He was feeling well and insisted he must go home that day. But Dr. Harris said that he should stay in the hospital one more night. Juan Carlos was upset. With wide steady-eyed impudence, which contained the threat of defiance, he glared at Dr. Harris. A scowl appeared on Dr. Harris's face and it deepened as he listened.

"I've got things to do tonight," he said, gazing earnestly out the window.

I figured that Juan Carlos was bored lying there in the bed with nothing to do. But Dr. Harris, who knew better, said in a hollow tone, "He has a score to settle and won't rest until he settles it."

I gave no answer except a sigh, which escaped involuntarily.

During the evening rounds, I went to the nurses' station on the pediatric floor and looked for Juan Carlos's vital sheets. They were nowhere to be seen. I asked an attending nurse. Her nonchalant reply stunned me: "He's no longer in the hospital."

"Why? But why?" I asked. "What do you mean he's no longer here? Dr. Harris didn't want him discharged today."

"We didn't discharge him; he took off."

I ran down the hallway to his room, but Juan Carlos was not

lying there in his bed. The white sheet was speckled with a trail of blood leading to the catheter tip dangling from the IV pole. He had pulled out his own IV and fled.

It was a Friday night, when the hunters and the hunted meet in the violent streets of a crime-ridden city. Brought to a standstill at the foot of the blood-splattered bed, suddenly, involuntarily, I rooted for Juan Carlos. I hoped this time that he would be the hunter.

FOURTEEN

BY *Tony Dajer, M.D.*

he ambulance call had come ten minutes earlier: suicide attempt, a hanging. I stayed in my easy chair — the unflappable ER doc. Besides, prisoners at the local jail were always stringing themselves up with bedsheets. Good way to spite the sheriff. And one reason they build jail cell ceilings low.

The emergency room doors slammed open. A squad of paramedics stormed in. Within their phalanx came a body jouncing limply on a stretcher. Then I caught a flash of blue. It was the face, glowing as blue as radioactive cobalt. Fourteen, they said. The girl on the stretcher was fourteen years old.

"They couldn't tell us how long she'd been missing, Doc," the chief medic told me between fierce, unnatural strokes to her chest. "In the barn ... grandmother found her ... long leather belt strung over a ceiling crossbeam." He straightened and wiped his brow. "Looks like she jumped off a concrete dividing wall." His gaze shifted to a point several feet behind my shoulder blades. "The wall was high."

He shook his head as if to blur the image of her body leaping into space to meet the fiercely sought, final unimaginable snap.

Fourteen. How did Shakespeare know to create Juliet a fortnight shy of fourteen?

Lovingly, the nurses slid her from the stretcher to the resuscitation table. The girl's face already seemed shrouded, too quickly darkening for me to see clearly. Only her eyelids lolled open, revealing the ground-glass murkiness peculiar to newly dead corneas. Even the yellow light of her well-moussed hair couldn't penetrate the penumbra settling over her features like mists on a lake at twilight. Out of her mouth, dangling like a dead steer's tongue, came the tube the ambulance medics had inserted into her lungs. One of them squeezed rhythmically on the attached plastic cylinder, forcing oxygen into indifferent lungs. But the neck was the worst. While the face was dead, the belt burns — angry and jagged — glowered beneath her chin like hot coals.

"Strip her," I heard myself command. This was a trauma code after all. There might be other injuries. Years of medical training nurture a holy restraint of the power that gives you the run of a female body — and bring a loathing, a howl of sacrilege, against any who violate it. "Strip her," I'd ordered, and suddenly wasn't sure why.

The nurses in that little rural emergency room were very good. They had her clothes off and two IV lines going before I'd even asked for adrenaline and the shock paddles.

Now the girl's body lay defenseless under the surgical lights. She was gorgeous. Her skin, smooth and tawny, glistened with a young girl's flawlessness. Her womanly breasts rose into nipples still pale from puberty. Her flanks swelled into hips and thighs made taut by a farm girl's life. How would that body look, I wondered, clasped in a boy's arms, riding waves of lovemaking? Where in that anatomy, where in that full-flowering form lay the death wish?

And how long, it suddenly struck me, had I been staring?

"Adrenaline, one ampule," I barked. A young heart has to be deprived of oxygen a long, long time before it goes flat-line. But maybe beyond the sensitivity of our electrodes something flickered.

TONY DAJER, M.D.

106

Resuscitations generate a camaraderie as pure in purpose as in function. Like trapeze artists who know exactly where to reach for a partner's waiting grip, the nurses and I could link up at breakneck speed to brake onrushing death. But now there was no anticipation, only a mechanical response to my orders. In between they kept their arms crossed tightly: whether in doubt or judgment I couldn't tell.

"Paddles!" I pressed one hard against the girl's upper sternum, the other against the roundness of her left breast.

"All clear!" I hit the discharge buttons. Her chest arced off the table. But her arms and legs hung back flaccid, like jaded observers of an old science-fair trick. The monitor tracing stayed flat. Her eyes kept staring at their own opacity.

I was ten when I saw my first dead body. My sister burst into the house, sobbing. Down the street, a little boy had fallen into his aunt's pool. My buddies and I jumped on our bikes and raced over. Through the picket fence around the pool we could see a small form lying under a white sheet. A pair of shoes, black and schoolboyish, protruded; the toes pointed upward to form a V. Only a policeman stood by, scratching in a notebook. The summer sun beat down. No clouds closed in to mark the boy's passing. No sobbing sounded. It felt like a stadium, empty and huge. Back at my house, we tried to calculate whether the shoes counted as a real dead body. Well, one of my friends argued, we *had* seen the body's outline under the sheet. We held on to that image like a trophy won at some personal peril. But none of us cried like my sister.

The adrenaline and the shocks weren't working. I should have called it off but I ordered cycle after cycle. I needed to keep impersonating a doctor the way an eclipse watcher needs to gaze through smoked glass to keep his retinas unscorched.

"Central line, please." The head nurse handed me an unnatural, vicious-looking needle with a catheter threaded through the bore.

"Last resort," I reasoned out loud: Pump adrenaline directly into the heart. I poured iodine over the girl's left collarbone, then stabbed beneath it. As I worked the needle upward I noticed, again, how impossibly smooth the skin on her chest was. She kept pulling me in, a whirlpool of beauty and death. A jet of bright red filled the catheter. The gloaming blue of her face mocked me. We pushed our adrenaline into her heart, but it had died with her leap.

I took my hands off her and stepped back, pulled off my gloves speckled with her blood.

The nurses turned her over, grappled with her legs to insert a catheter so we could run a pregnancy test on her urine. One of the medics produced the suicide note. The head nurse and I read it.

A boy, of course, and her father who hated him.

"No spelling mistakes," I heard the head nurse say softly. Then she looked up, surprised to have said such a thing.

The note, at the end, dispensed farewells and forgiveness like garlands (did I leave anyone out?), for once without fear of their being dropped.

The pregnancy test was negative. She had flung herself off that wall not to escape, but to punish. I wondered if after the first horrific check she had stayed conscious, slowly suffocating. Or whether the light had gone out in one final startling moment.

Out in the hallway stood a skinny, tattooed man wearing a cutoff T-shirt. His head, like a wayward churchgoer's forced genuflection, bent into the shoulder of a cigarette-wrinkled woman. Father and grandmother. No waves of grief surged from them — just a sense that they'd better hold this position until someone told them what to do next.

Back in the resuscitation room, the nurses were quietly picking up.

TONY DAJER, M.D.

"Thanks, everyone. Good job," I said without meeting gazes.

At that moment, the girl's body shuddered. A large brown stool pushed itself out from between her thighs. The nurses rushed to clean up the mess. That done, they set her legs out straight, tucked her arms against her sides, and wrapped her from head to toe in a new white sheet.

As if to convince me, finally, that all that was left on that resuscitation table was a corpse.

MECHANISM OF INJURY

BY *Hamish MacLaren, M.D.*

When you are a student in medical school, well-meaning professors (some of whom I suspect have not spoken to a patient in ten years) lecture you about the importance of taking a good History. "By the time you have taken the History," they cry stentoriously, "if you do not have an idea of the diagnosis, then you probably never will." So damn smug, those academics.

"It's the law of diminishing returns. History . . . examination . . . investigation. The subsequent steps are less and less useful to reaching a diagnosis if they are not established on the solid bedrock of an accurate History. And don't be tempted to call your patient a 'poor Historian.' Remember, it is the person writing the account down who is the Historian." I wish I could jerk this pompous professorial twit from out of his cloister into my emergency room and introduce Mr. Walter Burrows.

He was a small, wiry, bright-looking chap in his mid-fifties, smiling and holding up the remains of his right hand, wrapped up in a bloody rag.

"What happened, Walter?"

"It's me hand, Doc."

"Mmm. How did it happen?"

"I was gurning."

"Gurning?"

"Every working day of my life for the last thirty years I've been gurning, and this is my first accident. Bloody careless."

Well, it was an industrial accident of some sort. He was dressed in faded orange overalls and the bloodied rag was chamois. I ventured to say, "Gurning two days before Christmas?" still not having any idea what he was talking about.

He grinned at me apologetically. "Time and a half."

"Whom do you work for?"

"Randell, Rendall, and Randell." I hadn't heard of them. I raised an eyebrow.

"A subsidiary of LMP." (Who the hell are they?) "Machining. Industrial supply."

"And what went wrong with the gurning?"

He warmed to the subject, even drawing diagrams in midair with what I suspected, under the stained chamois, to be a half-amputated hand.

"I was standing on a pallet on top of a fork-hoist, leaning on a graunching stanchion. Sometimes the gurney jams up on the mounting hooks. You're supposed to switch off before you free it up. I thought I could flick it over before the damping tamper came down, but I think there may have been a kickback. It all happened so quickly."

"Kickback?"

"Yes. You see it runs on pressurized carbon dioxide. You get kickbacks above two hundred PSI."

I had a vague vision of some nightmarish occurrence on an industrial conveyor belt. "Er, what sort of work do you do, Mr. Burrows?"

"Like I said, gurning."

"And what does the machine that you were operating do? What is its purpose?"

A look of puzzlement flickered across Mr. Burrows's brow, as if he were having to revise some notion that he had until then taken for granted. Was I the doctor, or was I a window cleaner in a white coat?

He said, hesitantly, uncertain that he was being asked to state the incredibly obvious, "It's a tamping gurney."

"Does it make something?" I felt as if I were taking part in some kind of game show. Is it something I could eat? Something I could wear? Would my friends envy me if I had one?

"No. It's a finishing process. Melding."

"Welding?"

"No. Melding."

"What do you meld?"

"Plant."

"You meld plant."

"You got it, Doc." He looked relieved. For a moment we stared at one another, in dead silence. I said, "Excuse me," and went outside. I took a few deep breaths. I don't know what possessed me, for I should have given it up there and then. Perhaps it was the memory of that sanctimonious professor. But I was determined to get to the bottom of this. I went back into the room, a moth attracted to bright light.

Perhaps if I concentrated on what happened at the tissue level. . . . I looked hopefully at Mr. Burrows. His eyes were bright and clear, honest, candid, trusting. From the depths of my subconscious, I heard my ancient professor saying, "Ask open-ended questions. Never ask leading questions." I said, suppressing that noxious voice, "Did you crush your hand between two heavy plates?"

"No, not exactly."

"Did it get sucked in?"

"Nope."

"Was it a direct blow?"

"More sustained than that."

"Like a crush?"

"I'm not sure that crush — "

"Or a torque?"

"I lost my balance — "

"Was it a FOOSH injury?"

"FOOSH?"

"Fall on outstretched hand?" I can get technical, too, Mr. Burrows. You aren't the only one round here with idiotic jargon.

"Not really outstretched . . ."

"Twisting? Pulling? Pushing? Traction? Avulsion? Traction-avulsion? High pressure–high velocity? Explosive?" But nothing on the menu appeared to satisfy Mr. Burrows, nor exhaust his patience. I began to feel like an irate Los Angeles district attorney. "Your Honor, request the court's permission to treat Mr. Burrows as a hostile witness." The judge, a big black man, would have had a disconsolate expression, as if he had just sucked a lemon. "Dr. MacLaren, I'm going to allow you some latitude here, but keep it brief."

But Mr. Burrows would not be broken, and his gaze remained unaverted and unblinking. There was silence. I said, "Excuse me," and left the room.

Outside, I bumped, literally, into the nurse. "Pattie. Do you know anything about graunching tampons?"

"I beg your pardon?"

"Never mind."

Back to the fray, the vertiginous drawn to the precipice, the explorer caught in the quicksand — the more he struggles, the more he is sucked in. I had one last inspiration: the power of mime.

"Mr. Burrows, do you think you could show me how you did it?"

Mechanism of Injury

"Sure, Doc. It was like this." He stood up too quickly, and turned pale. "Oh, I'm feeling a bit faint!"

"Nurse! Pattie!"

I sprang up, caught him as he slumped forward, and led him a few faltering steps to an examination table. I maneuvered his head and trunk to a supine position, with his legs still on the floor. It was a bit like dipping a partner on the dance floor. Pattie finally entered.

"Yes, Doctor?"

I brought the legs in the faded orange overalls up onto the exam table. The skin I noticed was clammy, the overalls a little damp. "Would you mind taking Mr. Burrows's blood pressure? He's just feeling a bit faint." I finally came to my senses. Enough of this Historical nonsense. Time to perform an examination, get an X ray. I stepped out into the corridor again. There was something about Mr. Burrows that I could take only in small doses. Pattie was tut-tutting about the puddle of blood on the floor leading from Mr. Burrows's chair to the table. She took the cuff of the sphygmomanometer down from its position on the wall.

Two men were approaching down the corridor from Reception. They were dressed in orange overalls identical to Mr. Burrows's, and I noticed that one of them was carrying a transparent plastic bag half full of ice.

"Is that . . . " I pointed. "Mr. Burrows?" The younger of the two men nodded and grinned toothlessly. It had perhaps been an unfortunate way of putting it. I took the bag. "That's excellent. You never know; it may come in useful." A sudden, last despairing try. "Did you see it happen?"

"Oh, yes."

"What did he actually do?"

The two men looked at one another, muttered something inaudible, appeared to reach agreement, then turned back to me.

" 'Caught his hand in the rotor arm of the stent gun," said the younger man. He had a lisp. I stared at him, thinking, You really have a terrible dental problem. You ought to go see an orthodontist.

I said, "You mean it wasn't a kickback on the tamping gurney?"

He smirked. "Same thing, Doctor."

I said, "Thanks. You've been a great help," and went off to deposit the rest of Walter Burrows in the fridge. And to this day, I have no idea how Mr. Burrows came to injure his right hand.

DISCOVERIES

BY *Stewart Massad, M.D.*

She might have lied. She might have sent him out. She might have said nothing; pain gave her that privilege. But in the end the husband always finds out. With me there, her gynecologist, he had to stand and listen.

Myself, I'd rather have missed her story. I should have been home, and it was much too late for a normal guy to be working, but normality's never been one of my vices, and no one was waiting up for me. Besides, I had a patient upstairs, a high school junior with a few hours of labor left to make the transition between childhood and motherhood, so when I got the call from the doc in the emergency room about a woman with belly pain, I went.

The husband jumped up when I opened the door. He was a smooth guy in a double-breasted suit with a little mustache and a case of nerves. I introduced myself. He pumped my hand. She just looked up and nodded, then went back to rocking herself on the end of the examining table.

She was one of those women who dress up before leaving for the hospital. Unlike many, she hadn't overdone it: a little powder, lipstick in an understated shade, clear nail polish. Her brown eyes set off red highlights in long blond hair pulled back with a black ribbon to show off earrings that matched her wedding band. It looked nice, but it all made the hospital gown look even more shabby than usual, and not even house paint could have hidden her pain.

She was bent over, arms around her middle: the classic posture of peritonitis, almost good enough to hang a diagnosis on. The pain was not so bad, though, that she couldn't smile when I introduced myself, put a hand on her shoulder, and promised I'd take care of her. Hers was a soft, quiet smile, wholesome and hopeful but brittle as glass.

On the clipboard that was all she had for a chart the triage nurse had circled her temperature, in case the number 103 didn't catch my eye. Her pulse was quick, but her blood pressure was strong enough that we could work through the diagnostic questions I'd known since medical school rather than rush to the empirics of resuscitation. She was twenty-six, married, a photographer. Her husband was a lawyer. She'd had her appendix out halfway through the second grade. She didn't smoke, drank only socially, used no illicit drugs, took no medicines, was under no doctor's care.

"Birth control?" I asked her.

The husband broke in: "We've been trying for a baby since Christmas."

He was glowing at the thought, the prospective family man. She did not look at him in contradiction, only answered in a voice just loud enough for us both.

"I'm on the pill," she said.

She looked not to him, but up at me: for sympathy, maybe, maybe for forgiveness, maybe for reproach. The husband opened his mouth to say something. Instead he frowned, sat uneasily back against the wall, and bit his mustache. I, who knew neither of them, just nodded, dropped my eyes to the notes on the clipboard, and went back to my questions.

She'd been fine until the end of her last period, when she'd first started to notice pain, thought it was cramps, and done nothing about it. She had a little discharge, then a little pain with intercourse on Sunday morning. Over the last two days, the pain had grown so she could only walk hunched over. She'd tried Tylenol, Advil, Bufferin, even a couple of Percocet left over from the spring she'd had her wisdom teeth out. Nothing had helped. She'd waited till her husband came home before coming in. After all, he was a junior partner, worked every night till nine, was charging hard through the corporate ranks. She'd been afraid to bother him.

I kept questioning while I started her physical. The lymph nodes in her neck were fine. She had no tenderness down her spine or over her kidneys.

"Cold stethoscope," I warned. I took the cotton blanket off her shoulders. She shivered. She had fine, white body hair in a line along the trough of her spine, supple muscles under clear skin, breasts that pregnancy had never stretched. She had a runner's heart and lungs, did four miles each day along the river and past the high school. She had not been out in four days, a measure of the pain she'd been neglecting.

The conversation lagged. "Been married long?" I asked.

She smiled, remembering, then glanced at him. "Seventeen and a half months."

I nodded, remembering my wedding, fond retrospection colored through the lens of divorce.

I pulled out the footrest at the end of the examining table, and she lay back gingerly, her knees coming up involuntarily to guard her belly. When I pushed near the pelvis, she winced, and when I took my hands away, she cried out. It was a short cry, bitten off in shame.

I went out to get help with the gynecologic exam. The husband followed: No man, I suppose, wants to watch another's hand inside his wife's vagina. I did not wait for him.

"How is she?" he asked, catching me at the nursing station. He had run a hand through his hair, and the little spikes done up so perfectly in styling mousse were all askew.

"She's in a lot of pain."

He didn't need a doctor to tell him that, but he kept his temper. "Will you have to operate?"

"Don't know," I said. I was busy reading the results of lab tests that had been sent off while I was on my way downstairs. She was not pregnant. Her urine was clean. Her white blood cell count was high.

We were running out of possible diagnoses. On the husband's young, unlined face, agitation and anxiety were amplified by ignorance. The orderliness of precedent and law was what he knew. In an emergency room, under the tao of chaos, he was lost. I had no reassurances. I left him.

In stirrups she eased down the table. She moved, one buttock at a time, with resignation and sorry anticipation, acceding to violation with a deliberateness that was its own protest. I put the speculum in as delicately as I knew, but she still whimpered. Opening the blades, I saw the pus all over everything.

I did the cultures and made myself a slide. There was no point to putting a hand in, she was so sore, but I did it anyway; her husband was a lawyer, after all. The inside of her vagina was feverishly hot. She pushed away.

"Oh, God," she said. As I took my hand away, she rolled onto her side to grip her belly, as if to hold in her pain, as if to hide it from me. Pain is such a private thing, after all.

I put a hand on the arm she had over her eyes. "It's okay," I told her. "It's a reflex."

She looked at me with wet eyes. "It's not that," she began. "It's . . ." Then she turned away.

The husband tried to stop me on my way to the lab, but I was in no mood. I heated my little slide over the burner there, put on the stains, washed off the excess. It was a cumbersome procedure, the Gram's stain. It is obsolete, replaced by DNA analysis and antibody testing. But it takes only three minutes. Under the microscope, the bacteria were there, little red biscuits back to back in sheets of pus.

I went back into the room and sat down. She was curled up on her side, watching me. She had her back to him. He was stroking one shoulder through the cheap gown, murmuring meaningless reassurances I could not hear.

"What is it?" she asked.

If it had not been so late, if I had not been so tired, if she had not been in such pain, I might have drawn out my answer, hedged it round with ambiguities and doubt. Instead, after I rubbed my eyes a moment, as if to rub out the unpleasantness that I knew would follow, I just gave it to them.

"It's gonorrhea," I said.

Since she knew, or at least suspected, she did not react. In fact, she grew quieter. She shivered, but perhaps that was the fever.

The husband, of course, took it differently. "Gonorrhea?" he said. He pulled away from her, took a step back. He stood alone in the far corner of the little room, boxed in by plain white walls converging. "Gonorrhea?" he repeated. "Gonorrhea?" As if repetition could make sense of the word.

"Yes," I said. I waited. She waited.

He blinked twice, as if to see how he should answer. He looked around the room. There was nothing familiar in it except his wife, and she was drawn up in a ball around her own hurt, no help to him. But he was a lawyer, after all, probably a good lawyer. He found himself in what he knew. He tried counterargument. "But we're married," he insisted. "And I haven't . . ."

He took his wife's hand, but though she did not pull away, the hand lay in his fingers as limp and pale as a wilted lily. "Honey, tell him," he pleaded. But she would not answer, would not look at him. In his confusion, he turned away from her to turn on me.

"God damn you," he said. "You've got a lot of balls, making allegations like that." He took a step forward, stabbing the air with one finger. "You don't know what kind of trouble I can make for you."

"I'm sure I do," I told him. I looked at him hard and straight and stopped him. I had been through this so many times before and always hated it, especially when the husband blames the messenger. "But that won't change what's on the glass in the lab."

Like street dogs we glared at each other a long moment. Then he folded his arms, gave us both his back. "Shit," he said.

From her I'd expected tears, but she was tougher than that. She glanced from him to me, but not at me. She just stared into the future, watching innocence dissipate with youth into the sterility of the air-conditioned room. She took a very long breath and slowly rolled onto her back. She gazed up at the fluorescent lights and asked me:

"Now what?"

I got up and put a hand on her forearm again. "You'll need antibiotics."

"No operation?" he asked.

"I don't think so."

"No hysterectomy?"

"No."

"You're sure?" she pressed.

I parried. "No doctor is ever sure. I don't think so."

"Do I have to go home, or can I stay?"

"You can stay," I promised.

I explained the importance of an ultrasound scan, intravenous drugs and fluids, frequent monitoring. I mentioned the child in labor on the fourth floor and my need to check on her.

I left them there together. They had much to talk about.

Upstairs the kid was doing all right. She was screaming with the pains, but she wasn't thrashing around much. And she was progressing — slowly, but still she was progressing. Her mother was not doing so well. I stayed until the epidural left them both quieter.

When I went back to the emergency room, my patient was still in the radiology suite. I cut through the CT-scan rooms into the ultrasound area. The place was lit up in blue and gray by the images on the ultrasound machine. The woman's tubes were pus-filled sausages, sealed by infection. I waited outside until the orderly took her back into the room.

She looked better, with the first dose of antibiotics on board, along with a shot of narcotics, a bag of fluids, and something for the fever. I put a hand on her forehead, a gesture my profs used to disparage but one I still use because my mother taught it to me. She was cooler.

She didn't wait for me to ask. "He's gone outside," she told me. "He wanted to be by himself for a while."

"I'm sorry," I said, though in fact I was not.

"He didn't take it well," she said, but then, no one ever does. She shook her head. "It's not your fault," she said, which was true. We let that hang in the air, and I remembered how little infidelities compound until the fabric of marriage tears apart. Then she shook her head again softly and focused us both on the case at hand. "How bad is it?" she asked.

I explained about the abscesses.

"I see," she said, though I could see she did not. There would be time later to discuss the complications of such bad infection: infertility, ectopic pregnancy, chronic pain. We were both tired.

"You'll be going upstairs soon," I told her. She nodded. "Only a few more questions. Have you noticed any sores on your genitals?"

"You mean like herpes?"

"Herpes, syphilis — "

"Syphilis?" Her eyes widened.

"I take it that means no."

STEWART MASSAD, M.D.

She shook her head vehemently.

"We'll be testing for it. It's a venereal disease. They tend to go together."

She was glum suddenly. "I see," she said. She was watching the wall, the unchanging shadows under the cabinets. "What else?"

"Ever been tested for AIDS?"

She closed her eyes. "We were careful," she protested. "He's not a — " But then she realized that she had not been careful enough, that there were things about her lover she hadn't known, hadn't even known to ask. Spontaneity, adventure, excitement, and love came layered with deception, betrayal, and lies, and they were all coming apart for her.

"You'll need to tell your partners," I told her. "They'll all need to be cultured and treated."

"My partners," she said. It was all so tawdry now. "God damn my partners."

She rolled over against the wall. It was a sign for me to go.

At the nursing station, I wrote out the admission orders, the history, the physical exam. I detailed our discussions, outlined the plan. When I was done, I went to the waiting room. The husband was not there. I went to the pneumatic double doors. He was outside, in the dark beyond the halogen lights under the awning, on the strip of grass between the ambulance parking and the visitors' lot. He was sitting with his head in his hands and his feet in the gutter.

GAMBLER

BY *John Lantos, M.D.*

I like driving home. We live in a predominantly black neighborhood. It's nice. Middle class. Doctors and lawyers like us. We must be one of the few white families in America to move to such a neighborhood. It may be on the way up or on the way down, I can't quite tell. I thought it was on the way up. A big bank opened a branch near us. They built some middle-income town houses around the block, complete with rolls of sod for the front yards. A new shopping center opened nearby. Things were looking good. But then the "For Sale" signs started popping up on our block. And they won't go away. Very bad sign. I should have seen it coming. Last year, when we refinanced, the assessor frowned when he looked at what we were claiming as the value of our home. That should have been enough. But we got the loan, and were lulled into a false sense of complacency.

Now I wake up at night and, among other things, worry about whether we'll ever be able to sell the house. Not that I want to move. I like it here. But I like the thought that I can move, that my house is salable, appreciating in value, that my net worth is going up, that I have something to borrow against. A cushion. I may not have that anymore. I may have made a big mistake coming here. I knew it was a gamble.

I lie awake and my wife snores beside me, mumbles something in her sleep. I listen to her steady breathing and breathe in the smell of her hair. I like it here. This is all I need or want, to live in this house until I die, curled close to the warmth of her dreams, breathing the perfume of her hair. I want to die like Joe will die, with a beautiful woman by my side. Joe has cancer. I'm his doctor.

People who are dying crawl to my clinic door. They come in herds, in droves, in flocks, they come in tribes, in clans, and, surrounded by loved ones, in big family sedans. They come in hope and fear, with checkbooks open and pens poised. They are desperate and hopeful, full of despair and clutching at straws. The more unassuming and self-deprecating I am, the more they idealize me. I offer them hope, in the vaguest of terms.

Although I couch the hope that I offer in the careful cadences of legalistic prose that my lawyers have written, they find it. They find it in the most unlikely places. I watch them read the long list of side effects and adverse reactions that are described as "possible complications" and I can see them thinking, Ahh, possible but not probable, not definite. It won't happen to me. My hair won't fall out, my gums won't bleed, I won't fill the toilet bowl with blood, or be left vegetative by a sudden and massive hemorrhage into my brain. I won't have intractable pain, my stem cells will take root again, healthy and nonmalignant, in the fertile soil of my bone marrow. I won't become aplastic, neutropenic, aphasic, hypotensive, immunocompromised, septic, viremic, fungemic. That stuff is only possible. It won't happen to me.

Like soldiers storming the beach, they imagine that the shells are fired for others, that they will scale the hills, destroy the enemy bunkers, march triumphantly into Paris, where girls will throw flowers from balconies and bestow kisses in the cafés.

Just tell patients the truth, they say. They have a right to know. But which truth? The truth of hope or the truth of despair? Joe White came to me and wanted health, wanted hope, and wanted the truth. Thirty-four years old, a barroom bouncer, black belt, railroad worker, single. No children ("At least none that I've heard about, Doc"). A girlfriend and a sister. Lung cancer. He came in with a cough. Thought he had the flu. Wrong. He was young and strong and so we blasted him with every rat poison, mustard gas, and roentgen ray that the healing profession has ever developed. But nothing we could fire at him was tougher than his little growths, his little sprouts, his bumper crop of mutated epithelial cells.

Now he was in the ER, writhing in bed, behind the curtain, still in pain in spite of a morphine drip giving him doses high enough to kill a horse. His head was bald and covered with scars from the herpes infection that he was just getting over. His sister was on one side, his girlfriend on the other, and he, in his narcotic haze, was insisting that I give him another round of chemotherapy, the newest drug, insisting that he was going to lick this thing. One of the girls painted his ulcerated tongue and lips with a lemon glycerin swab while the other adjusted his headphones and turned up the volume of the CD. That wouldn't be such a bad way to go. Turn up the music, dial up the morphine.

I like my job.

I have come to an understanding about death. We, my patients and I, have an agreement. We don't talk about death. There are others who talk about it. We know who they are. I have nothing against them. You want a referral to hospice, I'll arrange it in a minute, you can go gentle into that good night. But I offer something different. It is a silent affirmation of the value of fighting against the inevitable. I can tell the minute I look in someone's eyes whether they share it or not.

Look, most of my patients die. I don't deny it, but I don't accept it with resignation, either. I am a magician. Sometimes, the magic works. I don't know why. We talk about survival and death in percentages, as if those are scientific facts. Twenty-percent one-year survival. I don't know which 20 percent or who will be among them. But I know that each patient might be the one. And the patients who take those odds have a look in their eyes. They are the high rollers.

I like to gamble. On nights off, I head for the riverboats with a thousand bucks. I play craps. The green felt, the smooth casualness of the croupiers as they toss the chips my way or just as emotionlessly stuff hundred-dollar bills down the money holes, the memory holes, like so much garbage, so much compost. I like to watch people's faces as they hold the dice. Everybody is different. The black guy in a leather jacket, a Marlboro in his mouth, he squeezes a Jack Daniel's in one hand while he squeezes the dice together with the other, and he squeezes his eyeballs together, wrinkles his forehead. The man is devout, his prayer fervent and compelling. Hell, a black guy like him beat the odds getting here with a handful of hundred-dollar bills to gamble. The smart money would have him dead on a street corner.

Or the elderly couple, he in chinos and a navy blazer, she in a sundress and straw hat. They take turns rolling, discuss each bet. They kiss when they win and pat each other's hands when they lose.

I am nonchalant. I don't believe in prayer and I am here by myself. I will take whatever the dice have to offer. I know the odds, and I don't believe in luck. Sometimes I win a thousand, sometimes I lose that much. It means nothing to me. I make two hundred thousand a year. I'm gambling one day's pay. The odds are against me, but they're not so bad. I like the feel of the riverboat engines revving up as we make the turn at the end of the cruise out. On the ride home, ahead or behind, I go up on deck and watch the trees gliding past on the shore. I smoke a cigarette. I know the odds. I like to gamble.

My hospital is a shrine to progress. People go there to sacrifice themselves. Unlike some cultures, our ritual sacrifice involves vic-

Gambler

tims who volunteer. This is no Abraham binding Isaac. Isaac signs a consent form that has been approved by bureaucrats in Washington and personal injury lawyers here at home. Isaac pays for the privilege of offering himself up. He could, if he wishes, die peacefully at home, dreaming opium dreams. He chooses, instead, prolonged torment. In the end, he insists that we put a tube down his throat and attach him to a mechanical bellows, that we inflate his tumor-encased lungs with higher and higher pressures until his lungs pop like an overinflated bicycle tire. Then his heart will stop, and he wants us to send jolts of electric current through his body. If we offered, Isaac would probably ask us to rip open his chest and take his bloody heart in our hands and squeeze it and squeeze it. But we don't offer that. We are not barbarians.

What are my limits? What wouldn't I offer? I write the protocols, the algorithms. I decide who gets which drug and at what dose. I decide, in the abstract, who is too sick. I won't break the codes, I won't look to see who is getting drug and who placebo, who shall die by fire and who by ice. I won't play favorites, I won't load the dice. You come to my temple, you hold those dice in one hand like the other suppliants and you let them roll down the table. The odds are against you but the game is fair.

I didn't think I would be this kind of doctor. I always imagined that I would take care of patients with cancer, but I used to think that I would be humanistic, help them accept death. I thought that nobody would want this kind of care, that the doctors must be foisting it upon them. I found out that I couldn't keep people away. People flock to me like moths to flame. They want to immolate themselves. To them, I am light and warmth.

I got the call from the ER as I was driving home, through my integrated neighborhood, anxious about the "For Sale" signs. I went back. He needed me. I could only tell him that there were no more drugs to give, no more protocols to offer. He wheedled. He cajoled. He buttonholed the nurses, made them turn down his morphine and increase his agony so he would be awake when I came, awake and writhing.

"What do I have to do or say?" he gasped.

"There's nothing you can do or say, Joe." The last train has left the station and you missed it.

"I don't want to die, Doc. I still have things to do. I have to talk to my Dad one more time, I have things I want to tell him. He called me. He's coming."

"He's not coming, Joe. You said he was coming last time you were in, and the time before."

"He's been busy, Doc. He'll come this week. Keep me going for just a few more days, Doc, just a few more days."

"Nothing I do will help, Joe. It's futile."

"Do it anyway. I want to go out fighting. I'm not afraid of the pain."

I pat his hand, try to look sympathetic and walk away. I can't act nice anymore. I want him to die so I don't have to watch him suffer. I can't stand any more of his idiotic optimism. I don't have to do what he asks. I'm not a snake oil salesman. What if he asked me to cut out the cancer in his lungs, to amputate his legs, to ritualistically slaughter him? What he wants is insane, irrational, sadistic. He's trying to hurt me. He hates me.

I listen to country music as I drive through the dark city. I turn it up loud. Jilted lovers, murders, songs about Jesus. On the way home, I can't get Joe's face out of my mind. He reminds me of Nate Andrews.

Nate used to work for my parents. Odd jobs. He'd mow the lawn, rake leaves, shovel snow. Nate used to smoke and then, when he stopped, he took up toothpicks. He always had one in the corner of his mouth. He'd roll it around while he talked. Nate was a hustler.

He worked at Bethlehem Steel. He started at the blast furnace, worked his way up to foreman, bought a house in the suburbs,

Gambler

married, had a few kids. He was always ready to work for a few extra bucks.

One day, he came to rake leaves and he had a huge bandage on his arm. His wife had thrown a pot of boiling water at him. Scalded his arm. She'd found out that he was having an affair with a white woman. He laughed as he told me about it, how nice the white woman was, how he'd done anything for her, how much she loved him. You got the feeling the boiling water hadn't even hurt. He would risk everything for another night of that kind of love. I'd never seen Nate looking so boyish. He usually had a reticence, a suspiciousness. But not then; he looked as dreamy as a puppy after a good meal. But after a few minutes, I saw a sadness come into his eyes, too, like that scalding water had burned deeper than the blisters on his arm, had burned down into his soul, and he knew that he'd lost the gamble.

After that, we saw less and less of Nate. We heard rumors. Layoffs at Bethlehem, plants closing. His marriage fell apart. His teenage kids were in trouble with the law. I wondered what went wrong. He'd had everything going for him and thrown it away.

Our neighborhood is quiet and dark. I get home late. As I walk from the car, I hear a pop. A firecracker, or a small pistol? I go into the dark kitchen, the dog opens one eye and wags her tail, but doesn't get up. I pour a glass of J & B, take it upstairs. My wife is already in bed, dozing. I crawl into bed, she groans, rolls over and mumbles, "How was your day?"

"Okay," I say.

She drifts off. I watch the covers rise and fall. I like the way they drape over the curve of her hips. I finish my Scotch and turn off the light. We both have to get up early.

STUMP

BY *James Thomas, M.D.*

I t's been a busy though rather routine shift in the emergency room. I came on at eight A.M. and go off in twenty-four hours. I clear out the last of the patients and wearily head to the call room for a snooze before the cluster of early-morning chest pains inevitably arrive. As I pull the hospital sheet over my shoulder I glance at the digital clock on the desk — it's 2:58 A.M. The paramedic radio siren rudely jolts me out of bed: "Self-inflicted gunshot wound to the head . . . agonal respirations, no blood pressure . . . we'll be there in three minutes."

"No rest yet," I think aloud. Though I'm exhausted, there's no doubt in my mind that I can handle this case. After enough experience the treatment becomes rote. Still, it's tough to justify my caring for someone who clearly attempted to kill himself — especially at three in the morning. Maybe he'll die in the ambulance.

I walk into Major Trauma and run through my preparatory ritual. Lights on, get out my intubation equipment, turn on suction. May be bloody, so I put on a surgical gown and gloves. I hate getting soaked in blood.

I see the reflection of the flashing red lights in the hallway outside the room. The paramedics quickly wheel a cart toward me. Their faces are serious, ashen. I see a figure lying on its side; a young man. I can see curly hair on the back of his head. His right arm is at his side, his left up under his head.

"Blood pressure's 80, he's breathing spontaneously," the paramedic reports. They turn the cart around to transfer him onto a gurney. For the first time I see the front of his head. Nothing in ten years' experience prepares me for what I see. I'm tossed suddenly into a dream, a nightmare, a horror movie I know can't be real.

Where his face should be, there's a bloody crater. I lean forward to look, then instinctively retreat. I've heard about cases like these. A person puts a shotgun barrel under his chin, but angles too far forward. Instead of instant death, he blows his face off.

In horror I force myself to step forward. I'm an emergency physician, his doctor now, remember? I'm not supposed to let my emotional reactions interfere with the job at hand. But he wanted to die, didn't he? Is he breathing? Yes. I see his chest moving up and down. I make myself look at his head. I know the anatomy of the face but I recognize nothing here. No eyes, no nose, no lips, no tongue, just some skin hanging from the sides of the head. I think I see some teeth hanging three in a row at an odd angle. This is no longer a person but a hideously disfigured corpse. What do they want *ME* to do? He wanted to die, didn't he? This guy was so inept he couldn't even manage to kill himself. Hopefully, he'll stop breathing any second now and I won't have to deal with this any longer. He's lying very still, his chest slowly rising and falling. No one in the room says a word.

I jolt myself awake. "Let's start some IVs." Blood is slowly oozing from the hole in the front of his head, dripping onto the sheets beneath where it's collecting into a red pool, and then spilling onto the floor in front of my feet. I quickly thread two large IV lines into his forearms. "Get the lab. We'll need the routine work and let's type and cross six units of blood."

Everyone in the room jumps as the figure on the gurney lets out a barely audible moan. Could he be awake? "If you can hear me, squeeze my fingers." There's an unmistakable response. My mind reels. Not only is he alive, he's awake!

"Page the neurosurgeon on call, also Ear, Nose, Throat and Plastics. Tell them to come in." A nurse attending the rest of the emergency room leans into the doorway of the trauma bay from the hallway. "You've got a chest pain in bed one and a twisted ankle in four."

Suddenly he moans loudly and jerks his right arm up toward his head. He lets out a little cough as though trying to clear his throat. The nurse reaches for the suction but doesn't seem to know quite where to clear the blood from the hole. He lifts his head up from the table. "Lie back down, just take it easy," but not, "You'll be okay." He'll never be okay. If this guy thought he had problems before . . .

He's making another funny coughing noise, this time louder. He lifts his head off the table. He gags. He's about to throw up. Vomit spurts from the center of the bloody hole in the front of his head. In horror, the nurse and respiratory therapist jump back. This is becoming too hard to watch. I can't look anymore.

I go around to the back side of the gurney. "Take it easy, you're at the hospital, just lie still." I place two fingers in his palm. "Can you hear me?" Three squeezes — one, two, three.

My mind is swirling in all kinds of thoughts. Maybe I should make sure this guy doesn't make it. That may be the humane thing. If I could inject him with — Wait, that's irrational and immoral. But isn't that what he wanted? What kind of life can he possibly have now? He's got no face — no eyes, no mouth. Hasn't he lost the essence of his person?

Again he rears up, trying to lift his head. He wretches and vomits again. The smell is too much for the respiratory therapist; she quietly excuses herself.

The neurosurgeon walks in at that same moment. I'm standing alongside the cart, the patient facing away. I won't get vomited on from here, and I don't have to look at the front of his head. I study the doctor's face as he approaches. He's keeping his distance. He won't come closer than four feet to the head of the bed. His eyes look away, he turns and steps back. He turns right around and looks again. His face is contorted, stuck somewhere between revulsion and professional inquiry.

"He breathes spontaneously and squeezes fingers on command," I say.

"Well, then it's not a neurosurgical case then, is it?" Technically he's right, and besides, who can blame him for waking up at three-thirty A.M. to see something like this.

The patient's becoming more and more agitated. He bends his right elbow and points to the front of his head. He doesn't touch. He's trying to scream. It's a peculiar guttural type of noise. I think he's trying to say something over and over: "Ah, ka, ee, ah, ka, ii."

The ENT man is here. I watch him enter. He stops abruptly two steps from the patient. He tilts his head to the side and looks for a second or two. He steps back, then forward again, his face expressionless. He lingers a moment longer, turns, then leaves the room.

Now the patient is actively trying to sit up, moaning loudly. Jagged edges of torn skin hang surrounding the hole like a curtain. Every surface oozes blood. As he tries to speak, facial muscles twitch the skin, but there's no bony framework left and the skin jerks sickeningly up and down. He's fighting. "Ah, ka, ee . . . I CAN'T BREATHE." The nurse calls two cops in from the hallway outside to help hold him down. "Give him three milligrams of Valium IV, and get some morphine." I give him more Valium, more morphine, and more. It seems the more I give, the more agitated he becomes. He's shaking his head side to side, the limp skin hanging down and trailing behind, splattering blood everywhere. I leave the room to get some air.

JAMES THOMAS, M.D.

At the desk an orthopedist who's come in for another case offers some advice. "He's not gonna die, he's gonna live, and he's gonna sue you. He's gonna say it's your fault his face is gone and sue your ass off. Get pictures, lots of pictures."

I return to my patient and find four cops instead of two. I walk around to the face side of the cart. He's still lying on his side, struggling. Behind him the four cops, all dressed in blue, all standing in a row shoulder to shoulder, try to hold him down. I can't give any more sedation safely.

How long can it take for the operating room crew to get here? It feels like an eternity. The situation is a tough one to manage and all the consultants are out of the room. Where's the damn anesthesiologist? I walk back out to the desk to find the doctors sitting around in a circle discussing the case. "There's two lower teeth left on either side that you need to stabilize first. We could take some rib and — Hey, Charlie, how are you going to put him to sleep, anyway?"

Am I the only one hoping he'll quietly stop breathing over there in my major trauma room so we can forget this nightmare as quickly as possible? Maybe I'm so tired I'm not thinking clearly anymore. What about the patient, what does he want? Has anyone asked him? Is he capable of rational decision? Is he aware yet that his eyes are gone — that he'll be blind forever? That he can't smile? How will he eat? Will he be fed through a tube? Will he wait to regain enough strength to finish what he set out to do? Will he overcome it all and someday be an inspiration to others?

"Doctor, the chest pain patient's labs and EKG are ready." I go to see him. It's difficult to concentrate on his story. I walk back to Major Trauma. The cart is gone, the room empty. There's a puddle of blood on the floor. A red trail traces the cart's path down the hall, past my sleep room to the elevator and the operating room. I wearily head for the desk to sit down and complete the chart.

There, clipped to its front, is a California driver's license with picture ID. I look at the face in the picture; it's handsome, with a strong chin, dark eyes, full lips.

I go to my call room, shut off the light, get into bed. I realize I've been staring at the wall in the dark for fifteen minutes. It's 4:45 A.M. I close my eyes. The phone rings — it's the nurse.

"Doc, we've got a four-month-old with a temp of 104, and there's a guy with shoulder pain checking in out front."

And the beat goes on . . .

HMO, DSM,
GOODWILL TOWARD MEN

BY *Samuel Shem, M.D.*

Are you a psychiatrist?"

My guard went up, like an off-duty pediatrician is on guard around children. My shift was over, and I was walking out the door of Toshiba, the emergency unit at the big private mental hospital called Fireman's Pointe. A thin, neat man in a tweedy sports jacket and Woody Allen glasses stood before me. His eyes seemed tiny, small buttons, the kind you see on a baby's shirt. He was mostly bald, and his lips were sweet, pursed and expectant, a little pink heart. I nodded.

"My name's Nash. Mickey Nash. I think I need admission to this hospital."

It was my first year of residency in Psychiatry, which meant I had been taught the essentials of being a psychiatrist for five whole months. So I clicked on what I had learned was the first question to ask in any psychiatric interview, and as empathetically as possible asked, "Do you have insurance?"

"I have insurance. That's the problem."

"How's that the problem?" I asked, framing a Chief Complaint of "I have insurance."

"It's managed care, an HMO. 'Healthycare Incorporated.' Admission has to be approved by two doctors from the HMO, and none will return my calls. I've been trying all day. Most of the time all I get is a busy signal. The office is in Washington. State."

"Keep hitting redial."

"I do. When I do get through I get a secretary, never a doctor."

"Is it an emergency?"

"That's what the secretaries all ask. I'm not sure. It's certainly urgent. I'm thinking seriously of killing myself."

"How seriously?"

"I'm not sure. I have no standard of comparison."

"Tell them it's urgent. Be a little more self-assertive."

"You think if I say that, they'll get the doctors to call me back?"

"It's worth a try. Keep redialing."

"Thanks muchly, Dr. — " He read my name tag. "Shem. You're the first doctor who's taken the time to talk to me. I feel a little better already."

"Good." We parted.

It was the end of my first day in the emergency unit, the week after Thanksgiving. Emergencies in Psychiatry turned out to be a lot easier than in real medicine or Surgery. In Psychiatry there were only about six drugs that did anything useful — *if anything* — and the main decision with this Nash was whether to admit him or discard him back into the pack. And that decision was dictated not by reality, but by insurance. All that day, listening to the range of human foible and suffering of my eight admissions, I had felt increasingly excited. In terms of the people coming in through the doorway from the world, it had been exhilarating work; but in terms of the larger questions, it had been appalling.

The night before, Berry, my longtime woman friend, a clinical psychologist, had said to me, "Be careful, Sam. In Psychiatry, the period between Thanksgiving and New Year's is the worst."

"How's it the worst?"

"The holidays drive people crazy. It's the worst."

"It's the best! Our best time of year!" This was the other point of view. When I had walked into the emergency ward earlier that first day, Dr. Tom Heiler, director of emergencies, had said, "The best time of year for admissions! By Christmas, there are no empty beds. Empty beds mean stalled careers. When our beds are full, we profit."

He then introduced me to the emergency unit rituals. While he told me a great deal about the physical layout of the ward and the procedures for admission and the intricacies of the computers, he said nothing about the patients.

"What about the patients?" I asked, puzzled.

"The patients?" he asked, more puzzled.

"The *patients*," I repeated.

"Oh," he said, lighting up. "The *software*. What about it?"

"Will you be supervising me on them?"

Heiler stared at me, uncomprehending.

"Su-per-vis-ing?" I said deliberately, loudly, as if to someone who doesn't speak your language. "So I can learn about patients?" More incomprehension. "You know, *learn?*"

"Learn?" Heiler repeated, and then went on. "Emergency unit is short-term. After that, it's transfer further in, to inpatient unit. You better start. So long."

My first admission was a plumber named George, who told a horrific story. A few days before, on the way to Thanksgiving dinner at his parents' house, he'd glanced into the backseat at his laughing baby and plowed into another car. His wife and three children had been killed, "fried like eggs," he repeated, over and over. He denied being suicidal.

How could anyone keep on living with this? I wondered, and as I listened to him my heart twisted on its spindle, in pain for him, and yes, *with* him. For after four months with a terrific resident teacher named Lenny Malik I had learned that the most important action I could take with him was no action, but to really be there with him, listening, empathetically. And after my long year of internship and my year traveling around the world with Berry, I had learned that the crucial element in any healing — whether body or mind — is connection.

Soon George began to cry, and tears came to my own eyes.

Suddenly, Tom Heiler burst into the room and yanked me out into the hallway.

"You've been in there forty-three minutes," he said. "You can't take that long. These days, no health care provider can. Length of stay is down; beds are empty. Admissions are doubling every year, but the daily census is falling."

"But he's in real trouble, and — "

"You have seven admissions to do today by five o'clock. Seven, and we'll try to squeeze in two more, thanks to the runup to Christmas. The key to success here is to always stay one step ahead of yourself."

"But he's desperate. He needs to talk."

"Not now. Admit him. Talk to him on your own time, before eight or after five. You can't open things up on Admission. There's no time to work them through. Opening things up does more harm than good. Including physical exam and writeup, you should take fourteen minutes for Admission.

"Fourteen minutes? That's impossible."

"C'mon. I'll show you."

"But this guy is desperate. I'm getting a really good history."

"For Admission, you don't need much history. The girls on the phones in Pre-Admission get enough usually. The goal of Admission is to admit."

"But even to admit, I've got to think about him, about his treatment."

"We do no real treatment on Emergency. There's not enough time. Treatment is done on inpatient unit."

"Well then for diagnosis. I've got to give it some thought."

"Ah!" he said, as if solving a crossword puzzle. "*That's* your problem."

"Diagnosis?"

"Thought."

"What's wrong with thought?"

"Thought plays no part in diagnosis."

"You mean go more with my feeling?"

"Feeling?" said Heiler, really puzzled at this one.

"Feeling. What the patient feels, and what he makes me feel, what I feel with him. Affect." He stared at me uncomprehending. "*Go with the affect?*"

"No, not the affect. The decision. Don't think, decide. As soon as I stopped thinking as a psychiatrist, everything went a helluva lot better."

"But isn't thought essential in order to decide?"

"Thought gets in the way of deciding. If you think, you leave room for doubt. If you doubt, you can't decide. Like the college boards. If you put down your first impulse, the first shot out of the box, you usually got it right, right? If you thought, you doubted, and the other multiple choice answers started to look better and better, so you got paralyzed, right?"

"But this isn't multiple choice. There are feelings involved here."

"Take your feelings to your therapist. We don't do feelings here. Do you know how to make decisions?" I said I did not. "Decision tree algorithms. You get raw data from the patient. You look in the back of this." He held up a well-worn copy of a small, green book, the size of a child's first reader, the kind with the animals with real wool the child can touch. "*Quick Reference to the Diagnostic Criteria from DSM-IV.* You look in the back." He looked in the back. Sure enough there were many treelike charts, where you start at one branch and you come to a fork and decide which of those to go to, and another fork and another until you find yourself out on a limb with a single leaf and no more forks, which is diagnosis.

"The computer will do it all for you: diagnosis, medication, date of discharge. Let's go."

We went back into the room with poor George, who sat hunched over staring at a wall. "Hi there!" Heiler said loudly and cheerfully, and pumped his hand like a politician. "Mind if I ask you a few quick questions?" Before George could answer, Heiler was asking him a few quick questions.

It was astonishing. Starting with the Chief Complaint — "It's my fault" — Heiler would ask a question — "You feel guilt?" — and George would start to answer. Heiler was only interested in "yes" or "no" answers. If George started to explain, he'd cut him off with another question. At first they seemed to be talking at cross-purposes, but soon George got into the rhythm. Wanting to please his doctor, and perhaps feeling relieved that he didn't have to confront the painful feelings that had brought him into Fireman's, he barked back sprightly "yes" and "no," moving swiftly and neatly through the decision tree in the back of *DSM-IV* until his doctor smiled, rose, pumped his hand again, and said, "You have 'Mood Disorder, Major Depression, Recurrent, with Melancholia 296.33.' Your insurance will cover seven days in Fireman's. We'll start you on antidepressants. If we find you suicidal or psychotic, we will rediagnose you, and your insurance will cover more. Any questions?"

It looked like George had a lot of questions, but before he could start, Heiler was saying, "Thank you very much. Dr. Shem will do your physical. Have a pleasant stay in Fireman's," and was gone, dragging me along behind.

"Four minutes," Heiler said, proudly. "Have a nice day." He left.

I was appalled. This technique was the classic "medical model" I'd learned in my medical internship. Starting with a live human being, you asked a lot of trick questions to funnel the human down into a diagnosis and a treatment. You cut off conversation, for more talk meant less time for sleep. And yet Lenny Malik had shown me that being a shrink was doing the opposite: turning the funnel upside down, opening things up, in order to connect. "Drug companies and insurance tanks and the *DSM* slurpers want us to apply the 'medical model' to people's minds," he'd say. "But there ain't no pill you can give the soul." He'd shown me that connecting with people was delicate, meticulous, intuitive work, and after five months I finally felt I was getting the hang of it, unlearning most of my medical school training and my brutalization by my internship to —

"Hey, cowboy!"

My voice beeper. Viv, the telephone and beeper operator: "Admission number one's ready for his physical, and numbers two, three, and four are already here waiting for you, and number five is the Lady Who Eats Metal Objects and she ate her hairdresser's wedding ring and is on the way in, too, so don't think, honeypot, decide."

I did the physical exam on George. When I asked him if the scars across his chest where he'd cut himself with glass were attempts at killing himself, he refused to open up to me again and said, only, "Y'know, I really *liked* that guy, Doc Heiler. A real pro. Got straight to the point. You could learn a lot from him, y'know?"

When I went to do George's write-up, I found it already done, laser-printed and snapped into the chart. Heiler had given the computer the "yesses" and "nos," and the computer had given back a terrific Admission Note, with a medical model diagnosis of 296.33, which made poor George's catastrophe look as bloodless and manageable as any medical illness — though it missed the "glass mutilation, question suicide gesture," which I wrote in by hand.

Walking back to my other admissions, I resolved that I would never become that distant and cold and disconnected and technocrafted. It had happened in my internship and had almost killed me. I had chosen Psychiatry to try to learn to be human to sick people, and to be human in my own life. I would never let go of that vision, no.

I let go of that vision, quicker than you'd think. By Christmas the relentless pressures of the job — the need to admit more and more patients every day as insurance tried to discharge more and more patients every day — left no time for empathy. As I went through the emergency unit, day after day, week after week, each day closer to Christmas bringing in ever increasingly horrific human disasters, little by little, digit by digit, I gave in until I was playing five-digit *DSM* bingo on patients waiting to be admitted, and even on the people I cared for in my everyday life. The length of insured stay in Fireman's depended on the particular five-digit *DSM*; for a particular code the stay would be only three days, but for another, three weeks. Heiler had his finger on the pulse of the latest *DSM* diagnosis-payment roulette and would tell me, on a given day, what *DSM* the insurance would pay maximally for and would insist I use that *DSM*.

One day as I was heading off to the Fireman's Christmas party, I was buttonholed again by the Woody Allen lookalike in the tweed sports coat and tie, the man who didn't know how suicidal he really was and who was trying to get in touch with the doctors of his HMO — Healthycare Inc. — to certify his admission to Fireman's.

"I finally got through to a doctor!" he said, excitedly.

"Great. I knew your persistence would pay off."

"I said that if he didn't authorize my admission before the end of the year — next week — that I was going to kill myself, and that my lawyers were aware of this fact."

"Good thinking. When you mention lawyers, doctors start listening."

"That's what I thought, but then he said, 'You've been saying the same thing to our allied health professionals for several weeks now, and you haven't even made a suicide gesture, let alone an attempt. It doesn't sound all that much like an acute emergency anymore.' I told him that it was, but he said, 'I have to put you on hold.' I waited for almost half an hour, but he never took me off hold. Now what do I do?"

"Call back, start out sounding rational and then start screaming."

"Okay. Merry Christmas! Oh, God! — now I've offended you. I'm sorry."

"How have you offended me?"

"You're Jewish, right? You don't believe in Christmas."

"Who does anymore, I mean really?"

"Yeah." He squirmed and looked away, the way men do when they are about to try to make contact. "Dr. Shem, you're turning out to be my only friend."

It was the end of the Christmas season, and men were killing women and children at a brisk clip. On the morning of the last day of the year, the *Boston Globe* published a list of every woman and child killed by a man during the past year. It averaged out to one woman or child killed every five days. A woman had been killed every nine days. A child had been killed every fifteen days. Most men, after killing the women and children, killed themselves.

The last victims were the day before in a "safe" suburb, a family named Quist. Norman Quist first slit the throats of his two small children and dumped their bodies in a pond and then came back home and bludgeoned his wife, Colleen, to death. He then shot himself dead.

I had just admitted Colleen's sister, with a Chief Complaint: "I was the one who found my sister's body. Her head was split open by an ax and her brains were all spilled out and blood was soaking everything. Everywhere I go, I see her lying there, the ragged white of her skull, the dark blood, the pink brains. And he slit the throats of his children? They were angels, little angels. How can I live with this?"

When I came to giving her a *DSM* diagnosis, my mind got stuck. She wasn't crazy, she was what anyone would be: crushed. She needed time to heal, to be safe. The hospital wasn't a bad place to stay for a while, for her. But her insurance wanted her treated as an outpatient. I gave her the most innocuous *DSM* for which they would pay, "296.20, Major Depression, Single Episode."

I felt sick. Sick not only at the carnage, but at being a man. For most people who learn about killing by watching TV, the killing faded as quickly as anything on TV, basically gone by the next commercial and helped along to oblivion by the commercial itself, leaving no residue. But in Fireman's I had to live with the aftermath of the carnage, the enduring reality. What most people looked at from a couch as a flat run of pixels, *I saw*. Saw what it did to real live human beings, how it lasted not the six minutes to the next commercial, not six hours six months six years, but a lifetime. For weeks I had been having nightmares. I walked around enraged, sick at heart.

With one more empty bed, there were two on the waiting list:

The first was a Vietnamese refugee who, on finding his four-year-old daughter raped and strangled in an abandoned apartment, had flipped out, stalking the streets with a loaded .38, searching for Henry Kissinger. He was totally psychotic and dangerous.

The second was the head of a chicken franchise who was paying for hospitalization out of pocket who'd beaten his wife with a pool cue and had a Chief Complaint of "Why the hell was she putting on sexy underwear when we were getting dressed to go to court for our divorce, when she'd never wear sexy underwear when we were married?" He seemed pretty normal to me.

To whom would Heiler give the one remaining bed?

SAMUEL SHEM, M.D.

"They told us America is best country!" screamed the Vietnamese man as the security guard led him out the front door. ". . . they say you have chance. What chance my little girl have? I kill them all, you wait and see!"

I sought out the sanctuary of the bullet-proof cage of Fireman's Telephone & Beeper.

"Terrific," I said to Viv, the operator, taking her Christmas bottle of Chivas out of the bottom drawer and sipping. "We admit someone who is sane, and we send someone who is insane back out into the world. What's wrong with this picture?"

"Yeah, cowboy," she said, "it makes you wanna puke."

"Makes you want a law banning men from being around women and children."

"More bad news, Doc," said Primo, of Fireman's Security.

"Yeah?"

"They found a body, way, way back in the woods, frozen solid. And on the body was a letter and it was addressed to you."

He handed me a letter the size of a Christmas card. I opened it. A handmade Christmas card. Within a crude outline of a Christmas tree was written:

> Life is tough,
> Life is hard,
> Here's your fucking
> Christmas card.
> — Mandy

On the reverse side was a message for me:

Dear Dr. Shem,
My wife, Mandy, made me this card. You tried hard, but Healthycare kept putting me on hold. In my safe deposit

box is all the information, which our lawyer will use to sue the pants off Healthycare. My wife and kids will be taken care of. Thanks for your help.

Sincerely,
Mickey Nash

"You know him, Doc?"

"Not really."

"Died of exposure."

"Don't we all," said Viv, "in the end?"

"Yeah, well," I said, "we should give the guy a medal."

"Why's that, Doc?"

"He killed himself first. Before killing the wife and kids. This man was a great American. I'm off duty. Happy New Year."

I stared out the locked front door at the crowd, maybe twenty poor souls. Having been told there was no chance of getting in, the crowd turned nasty. Wild-eyed people were banging on the bullet-proof glass of the front door. How would I make it to my car?

Primo, the security guard, materialized to escort me.

We battled our way through, trying to stay on the sanded and salted walk, the crowd slipping and sliding on the ice on the lawn. It was pathetic, all these people sick of normal life, wanting into a hospital for the mentally ill. They were downstream from something. We were hauling them up out of the river, but nobody was looking upstream, for whatever that something was. And if there was an epidemic of violence and isolation in the world, well, there was an epidemic of violence and isolation in Psychiatry, too, with all these drugs, all these HMOs, all these *DSMs*, all these dead-hearted shrinks like me.

My car was blocked from backing out by a small nuclear family: father, mother, baby. The father came to my window and shoved a sign in my face: "Unemployed executive. Will work for food. Can you help?"

I thought of Malik. Once last summer, walking with him toward a sports store in the village, we'd passed a drunk asking for change. Malik had given him a dollar. I'd given nothing. The panhandler said to him, "Have a nice day," and to me, ominously, "and a *safe* day, you."

"Why'd you do that?" I'd asked Malik. "He'll just spend it on booze."

"It's just my way," he said, "of betting on the Divinity."

Outside my car window now, the man was jolted by his wife and baby. I started to dig into my pocket for change.

But suddenly I saw the children, all the children mutilated and killed by men, and though I heard Malik's voice telling me that these were cries from the mine shaft on behalf of us all, I was filled with despair. How could a God, something Divine, do this?

I looked at the man and shook my head no.

He gave me the finger and moved away, the harsh wind hitting him, sliding him back, his legs working hard to stay up on the ice and to keep his wife and baby up too.

The sun was a red teardrop in the notch of a mountain, leaving a darkness over our low hill. As I pulled away the klieg lights went on. The crowd seemed beaten down by them, shrinking back from the front door. Illuminated over the portico was a brand new piece of Fireman's, a roseate marble panel. Chiseled into it, in foot-high letters brought up ruthlessly by the artificial light, was "In Touch with Tomorrow. Toshiba."

"Exactly," I said out loud. "Better than being in touch with today."

A LONG WEEKEND

BY *Rod Hamer, M.D.*

The agents of New York Life, Lincoln Life, Prudential, and others furnished me with an endless supply of candidates for insurability. As a GP in town, I performed a number of such physicals each week. The exams were no-brainers, and though not enormously profitable, were sure-pay. The most important fallout from the exams was the fact that many applicants were new in town and had not yet aligned with a family doctor. So most would become regular patients.

Most of the applicants were complete strangers to me and since the insurance company's first question on the form was "How did you identify the proposed insured?," I usually asked to see their driver's license. This simple tactic had always gone without a hitch.

The third appointment of the morning was a New York Life insurance exam on Ralph Jamison, someone, Doris advised, I hadn't seen before. Mr. Jamison had arrived on time, been led to Room 2, and asked to don one of those synthetic gowns that made men look absurd. I entered the room about fifteen minutes late, fouled by the previous patient saying those perverse words, "By the way, Doctor, while I'm here would you also . . . ?" Just when I thought I was done.

Ralph Jamison, a forty-two-year old bantamweight, had the

aggressiveness and audacity of a rooster. Although a slight man, he exuded an aura of nastiness that won him instant respect, respect based on the fear that an explosion lurked at the interface of his personality and yours.

"Thought you'd forgotten me," he greeted me with another patient platitude that never failed to annoy.

"Really sorry about that, Mr. Jamison," I lied. "I know your time is important too, but this won't take long."

"These are asshole gowns. Ever put one on?"

"Er, no, I haven't, but you're right, they are kind of foolish."

"Ya know, your receptionist was chewing gum. Not very professional."

He was probably right as Doris had been reminded several times not to chew gum when there were patients in the office. I didn't approve either, but it was at least better than Ruthie in Dr. Ditmar's office who actually chain-smoked while working.

"Snaps the Dentine like a crocodile."

"Mr. Jamison, do you have some sort of ID, perhaps a driver's license? New York Life requires I identify you."

I awaited the next bevy of insults but they didn't come. Not yet.

He jumped from the table and went to a chair over which his pants were draped. Removing his wallet he then flipped through the series of plastic enclosures common to billfolds and stopped at the appropriate window. He thrust it before my eyes to read.

"May I take it?" I asked.

"All right! Take the damn thing!"

I studied the small DMV document, and because in those days there was no photo on it, I then made a brainless blunder, one that would exact a then-unparalleled emotional toll on me for the subsequent 120 hours.

My idea was to quickly find a picture of him, make the identification, and get on with the exam. Dimwittedly and without his permission I flipped the license window to another several down the line. What I saw, amusedly to me, was not a smiling Mr. J. but a heavy-breasted, naked woman whose tongue lasciviously protruded over her lower lip and from whose hairy pubic triangle presented a snake. Although it was over thirty years ago and my glance was for a period of milliseconds, I see it clearly today.

My photographic interlude was truncated abruptly as he catapulted to my side and ripped the lewd wallet from my grasp. In keeping with the serpentine theme he hissed like the proverbial puff adder, verbally attacking my mother and my DNA. I deserved the tongue-lashing and fully anticipated a physical one as well. He struggled for control of his fists.

Before I could blurt out an apology his vitriolic invective resumed. A volcanolike eruption belched forth, burying me in molten besmirches.

"No right . . . ," blah, blah, " . . . report to the AMA . . . peeping Tom," blah, blah.

By now he had ripped away much of the gown, but a shoulder and part of a sleeve had withstood his tearing, and he stood there, ludicrously in his undershorts, the garment fragment looking like a burn dressing of some sort. He dressed some, cursed some, and sometimes did both. A new barrage of damnations followed each piece of clothing or footwear put on.

"Mr. Jamison! You are absolutely right to be upset. I shouldn't have done that and I wasn't trying to be nosy. I'm really sorry. Would you like to reschedule?"

The slamming door gave answer to my question. Doris rushed in. "Are you all right? What happened?" Her gum was really snapping now. Like a crocodile, I thought.

The morning brightened after this catastrophe: a well-baby exam, an OB visit, a possible prostatic cancer, a suture removal, and, of course, a "tired all the time." The gamut, the lure of General Practice.

After lunch it was more of the same, including an uneventful insurance physical. No one was hostile. At four P.M., Mrs. Palmieri, a multipara, was admitted to my service at the hospital with leaking membranes and warm-up contractions. Dr. Holmdahl called just before six to sign out to me for the night. Ahead for me lay my practice, his practice, an OB starting to percolate, and ER coverage. Little did I realize that was the GOOD news.

The patron saint allowing doctors to eat uninterrupted meals bestowed his kindness and I had a rare Friday night dinner with my family. When had all those children come to live with us? My wife amazed me with her composure with the three tots and her ability to look so pretty while putting a meal on the table.

At seven P.M. I visited OB, and 5 centimeters of dilation discouraged my leaving the hospital. I went to Medical Records in an attempt to stem the flood of warning notices about delinquent charts. I had dictated three charts when the PA system ordered me to call the ER, but when I complied, there was a busy signal. Jackie, the PM supervisor who floated ER, was noted for marathonesque telephone conversations. If she was chatting, it probably wasn't urgent and I did a few more charts. As I tried to read some of my progress notes I was reminded of a chaotic ventricular rhythm, and interpretation was difficult. Then the phone nearby rang.

"Got one for ya. Pain in-the-ask-me-no-questions if I ever saw one," spouted the unambiguous Jackie.

"What do you have?"

"Forty-two-year-old jerkoff with a scalp laceration about two inches long and a foul oral cavity about two feet wide. Someone bashed him at Goldstein Motors. Going to sue everyone. Probably you, too. Get down here and sew him up. His cut and his mouth so we can clear him the hell out of here."

In passive-aggressive fashion I did two more charts and then strolled to the ER. When there I glanced quickly at the chart, noting only the Chief Complaint, "cut head," in Jackie's clear handwriting.

"Hello, I'm Dr. Taft. What happened to your head?"

"YOU," he screamed, sitting up abruptly and startling me. "Can't I get away from you? Peeping Tom! Dr. Quack! Don't touch me!"

It was *Jamison!* The man whose wallet I'd ransacked in my office. He sloshed his words, suggesting alcohol or trauma, most likely the former. I took his abuse for another minute and then interrupted him. "Mr. Jamison, you may be stuck with me, because I'm the only doctor in town on call for this ER. Do you have a regular doctor in town?"

"Hell, no. I've only been in town for two weeks. Why would I have a doctor?"

"If you prefer I'll try to get someone else to come in and see you," fully aware none of my colleagues would even answer a call from the ER on a Friday night. "The third choice would be for you to drive the twenty-five miles to the next city and get treatment there."

"Get someone else. I'm not driving twenty-five miles bleeding like a stuck pig."

I tried a couple of calls but had no luck. "No one is available," I advised him. "Let's call a truce and have me fix you. I won't even send you a bill. Consider it an apology for this morning."

"A bill? You think I'm paying a bill? That goddamn car sales-man will pay the bills. Besides, I'm suing his ass. The cops know he started it. Should have arrested him!"

"Who hit you?" I queried.

"The big heavy guy at the car place. Said I couldn't test-drive the piece of junk he was trying to sell me until tomorrow. Sucker punched me when I just tried to sit in it. My lawyer will clean him out!"

He was describing Al Epstein, a salesman who'd come to town two or three years before me. He was in his late thirties, a nice enough guy, but could have his fuse ignited at times. I had played softball against him twice in a slo-pitch league a summer ago, and in one game, Al, who caught, had a couple of close plays called against him at the plate. After the last one he had broken into a fury extraordinaire and he and the ump actually shoved each other. Jamison was an irritant and perhaps Al had decked him.

After humbling me in front of a nurse, an aide, a policeman, and a cleaning lady, Jamison backed off and allowed me to treat him. Although rabid, he was neurologically intact. Our proximity afforded me ongoing whiffs of his alcoholic exhaust. When I anesthetized the short, sharp-edged wound, he vehemently rejected my description of a "tiny bee sting." Four sutures, a refused tetanus booster, and we were done. This incident was long before the computer produced instruction sheets patients sign today, but he was given verbal head injury– and wound-care instructions. I went elsewhere to complete the chart.

The rest of the night was even busier and I was an irritable, sleep-deprived dispenser of care at Saturday morning office hours. We were finished just before noon and I began writing some overdue checks when the ER called.

"Doctor, I know you're off ER now," apologetically began Lorraine, the daytime weekend RN, "but the police just brought in a DOA and they want someone to pronounce him. Dr. LaVoie is on call for the ER but is in the OR with a bowel obstruction and Dr. Paige is with him and their third partner is coaching his son's swim team at the pool. Be a dear and come by and do it. I'll make it worth your while sometime."

She had used that ploy before but never had lived up to it. She was at least sixty-eight.

I wrote two more checks, probably dropping my unbalanced account perilously low. A small-town perk is an understanding bank officer. The phone rang again and a very serious-sounding policeman briefly identified himself and got my rapt attention with a sobering revelation. "I'm at the hospital with the DOA. The deceased is a Ralph Jamison, the man whose head you fixed last night, the one in the altercation at Goldstein's. He was staying at La Purissima Motel and a maid found him dead on the floor in his room this morning. We need you to get here as soon as you can."

I had never received any news that scared me more. No doubt I'd missed a developing epidural hematoma or some other intra-cranial disaster. Maybe someone had murdered him. I admit I briefly hoped so.

At the ER I examined the deceased. No doubt, it was Jamison. His nakedness in death made him appear smaller than before but he was still easy to dislike. The only external evidence of disease or injury was the sutured scalp and an ecchymotic area around his right greater trenchant. I formally pronounced the obvious and sat down with two officers. I told them the entire story.

"Well, Doctor, here it is in a nutshell. From our perspective your involvement in this is essentially nil. You aren't a suspect of any crime and other than getting your statement clarified a bit we won't detain you. From a medical malpractice point of view, well, that's another thing altogether. If he died as result of the head injury, you could have a problem. Possibly a large one. Maybe you should talk to your attorney. Off the record, strictly between us, Al, the car guy, could be looking at a manslaughter or worse charge. I mean, if he died from the blow. Coroner Creighton's away till Monday and I guess he'll do the postmortem then. That autopsy will be very important to both of you. Sorry, Doc, it's going to be a long weekend."

It already had been.

At home I tried to sleep but shame and fear kept me awake. I couldn't even bring myself to tell my wife what had occurred. Finally I decided to drive to the ocean and walk the shore, a generally tranquilizing experience. My route took me past Gold-stein Motors and almost reflexively I made a U-turn and pulled into the parking area.

The "Closed" sign was up but through the plate glass I could see Al Epstein's head bent over a desk. He was startled by my rapping but came to the door. It was probably poor judgment for me to have approached him but it was too late now. When he opened the door his reception implied he wanted to talk as much as I.

"The little son of a bitch pushed me too hard, too far. He was yapping like a terrier, trying deliberately to provoke me. He had been looking at a 'sixty Falcon Wagon with sixty-five thousand tough miles on it. Asked a million questions. Criticized everything about the damn car. Tires were too thin, lighter didn't work, plates rusted. Said we'd probably turned the odometer back twenty thousand miles. Smelled like a brewery and acted half drunk. Wanted to test-drive it in his condition! I tried to tell him in a polite way he shouldn't be driving anything and asked him to come back tomorrow. That really fired him up. Called Abel, the owner, a kike. I told him to watch it 'cause my name was Epstein. Then he raved about Nazis having the right idea. He couldn't seem to drop it, just steamrollered with all these insults. I lost it and grabbed him by the shirt with both hands but he was a strong little prick and yanked away from me. His pull sent him backward and he fell against the car with his butt and then veered off to the left. That's when he smacked his ugly head against the bumper edge. All I did was grab him and he's dead!"

He continued. "I tried to help him up but he spit at me and got himself up and stumbled to his car, bleeding all the while. He was calling me every name in the book and claimed he'd ruin me financially. I didn't know what to do! Just as he drove off another customer came in and I had to talk with her for what seemed like forever. After she left, the police came and well, you know the rest. I could kill that little bastard."

"You already may have," I commented.

We commiserated for another half hour. He was terrified and I wasn't much better off.

"We could both go down the tubes, you know," he told me. "Have to wait till Wednesday to find out. That's what you call a long weekend."

"Wednesday?" I shouted. "What happened to Monday? They said the coroner would be back on Monday!"

"They were wrong. Someone double-checked and found out Creighton is away till Wednesday. He's in San Fran stuffing his face at the Wharf or the Top of the Mark while we sweat blood here. Maybe the evidence will rot by then."

Al was partly right. Bodies, human or otherwise, are always just a couple equations away from rotting. One missing enzyme or substratum and we're garbage. But Ralph Jamison wouldn't be compost in four days. Unenthusiastically we shook hands and wished luck, but self-preservation rules. I knew that Al secretly hoped that I was the guilty one, and I, he.

The next few days were rough. I reviewed my meager financial resources and readied for the worst. A malpractice case would pummel my image and practice. Although I had some insurance, if I lost, it would not suffice if there was a major award. Jamison must have had a family of some sort since he was trying to get life insurance. I received perverse pleasure in knowing that his anger with me and not completing the physical would deny his estate the ten thousand dollars he applied for. At least New York Life was off the hook.

This personal crisis preceded the Cuban missile one by a few months. Since then I've had a few others, some more serious than this, but this was the first and I took it like a melanoma. An ominous sense of dread pervaded my thought and only occasionally was buffered by a few hours of sleep or attention to a patient's complaint. At last, Wednesday, Wednesday.

I was there for the autopsy at eleven A.M. Dr. Creighton must have enjoyed the city by the bay because he laughed and joked throughout the dissection. "Don't worry, I've been sued before and the sun still rises," he reassured.

"The body is that of a sixty-four-kilogram, one-hundred-sixty-five-centimeter Caucasian male," he began, speaking into an overhead mike.

He addressed every conceivable minutia, prolonging my wait. I had hoped he would go out of order and do the head first but he did not, staying in protocol. He may have been jocular but he took his job seriously.

Then, seemingly hours later, I heard him record, "And the anterior descending branch of the left coronary artery contains a large premortem thrombus," and later, "The cranial cavity is smooth and both the epidural and subdural spaces are clear. The entire cerebral cortex appears atrophic for age."

Then finally, "Probable cause of death is coronary thrombosis."

Jamison had died a cardiac death, a myocardial infarction with a probable fatal dysrhythmia. Half an hour later I was in the office removing stitches from another scalp wound.

BRING THE BOTTLES

BY *Tom Janisse, M.D.*

C arla handed me her initial assessment of the next patient, Mr. Reiz, a sixty-three-year-old man accompanied by his wife of approximately the same age. She was concerned that he appeared quite distressed, though didn't look seriously ill.

Mr. Reiz appeared clean-shaven, with short hair where he still had it on the back and sides of his head, somewhat overweight, showing most in his round face, double chin, and protuberant belly. His plain turquoise shirt was buttoned at the neck. Mrs. Reiz sat on the edge of her chair, knees together, purse in lap grasped by both hands. She wore her graying hair pinned up in a bun, and her apricot blouse had a floral pendant fastened exactly even on the left collar tip.

"Hello, Mr. Reiz. I'm Dr. Janisse. And you're Mrs. Reiz?"

"Hello, Doctor — "

"Hello, Dr. Janisse, yes, I'm Mrs. Reiz."

"What seems to be the matter, Mr. Reiz?"

"Well, Doctor, I — "

"Doctor, he hasn't been feeling himself. Have you, Joe?"

"No, Doctor, last night — "

"He was nauseous, didn't eat his normal supper. Not even his mashed potatoes!"

"Nauseous?"

"You see, Doctor, I just had — "

"His left kidney removed. Two weeks now. He's been doing real well. Haven't you, Joe?"

"Have you had a fever, Mr. Reiz?"

"Yes."

"Yes."

"When did it first go up?"

"_____"

"Joe, when?"

"You tell him, Lilly."

"Last night. It wasn't much, but this morning it really shot up. That's when you had the chill. Right?"

"Yes, I believe I did have a chill. Shaking like."

"Anything else, Mr. Reiz?"

"Well, that's when I threw — "

"Up. His whole breakfast. Not like him. At all. Eggs, bacon, biscuit, grits, juice, coffee. In fact some of it didn't even look eaten."

"How do you feel now?" I asked.

"Tired. He's got no life in him."

"Honey!"

"Yes?"

"Please let me answer the doctor's questions. He's asking me. I'm the one that knows. We agreed on this before we came."

"Yes, okay, I forgot."

"Doctor, I'm feeling kind of tired. Not bad really. Got a little itching around this suture site."

"Does it hurt when I touch it?"

"No."

"Belly hurt here?"

"No."

"Over here?"

"No — "

"No. His stomach hasn't been bothering him. I'm worried about his . . . excuse me, you know, going to the bathroom."

"Yes, Mr. Reiz, have you been urinating more than usual?"

"Ye — "

"Yes, he has, as a matter of fact. Keeping me awake at night. Getting up several times a night. Makes me really tired and irritable in the morning."

"Does it burn, when you go?"

"Not especially."

"Oh, it does too, Joe! You told me it did."

"Well, now that you mention it."

"Sounds like an infection in your urinary system that's causing this."

"Doctor — "

"Is that serious? He's a diabetic, you know."

"Shouldn't be serious. But if he's diabetic, we'll want to be sure and get on top of it."

"Good."

"Good!"

"Any other medical problems, Mr. Reiz?"

"Well, let's see, I do have — "

"Gout. It's better now that winter's passed."

"Lilly, please."

"Well, Joe, you don't always tell the doctor all these things. You forget. He has to know."

"Mr. Reiz, what medicines do you take now?"

"_____"

"Any?"

"Doctor, you'll have to ask my wife. Lilly, can you — "

"Here, I have the list right here. I wrote them down so I wouldn't forget. At a time like this. I told you to bring the bottles, Joe."

"I don't pay attention to those things, Lilly."

"Well, you should. Look here. Here's the list, Doctor."

"Thank you."

"Doctor, do you think I'll have to have surgery again?"

"No, Joe, it's only a bladder infection. I've had those. You just take some pills."

"But I threw up this morning. And my stomach doesn't feel that great. I don't think I can take any pills."

"That's important," I said, supporting him. "We may have to keep you in the hospital until things settle down, what with your recent surgery, fever, vomiting, diabetes, gout — "

"And his high blood pressure."

"Oh."

"See, I told you, Joe. To bring your pajamas. But no! Now I'll have to make a special trip home to get them. And leave you here alone."

"You didn't know, Lilly!"

"Let's check your urine and draw some blood. Then we'll put in an IV so you don't get dehydrated, and then we can give you antibiotics in your vein. Rest your stomach, and work faster."

"Okay."

"Good idea, Doctor. Joe, I knew that's what we should do. Best thing for you. Dr. Janisse, are you going to call his surgeon and tell him? He just had surgery."

"Yes, Mrs. Reiz. I'll do that. See if he'd like to do anything else. I think you'll be fine, Mr. Reiz."

"Doctor . . ."

"What is it, Joe?"

"She won't be able to stay in the hospital with me, will she?"

BLOOD ON THE TRACKS

BY *Tom Moskalewicz, M.D.*

Fred died during the year he was planning the date of his retirement. He had practiced Family Medicine in our community for thirty-five years, and he was leaving with good timing: still healthy and active, with plans to travel and to spend more time with his children and grandchildren. He was a good role model for us, and we told him so — an example of a physician who had given the self-sacrifice of long hours and many sleepless nights and still would be able to jump from the train with his health intact and ample time to enjoy the fruits of all his labor. We knew too many stories about other colleagues who had died shackled to the job.

Then the trauma of the unexpected altered his plans. On a clear, warming April afternoon, as he was walking with his two grandchildren, a freight train rattled around the bend and caught Fred in the center of an old wooden train trestle, high above a deadly river. A few seconds later he was knocked off it, falling forty feet into the swollen river, where he was swallowed up and carried away by strong currents. He left us without the opportunity to say a proper and respectful good-bye.

That Friday there had been dramatic changes in the weather. The morning blustered with sleet and swirling snow. By noon the skies had turned steely gray and the temperature had climbed to fifty. By four o'clock, as Fred set out on his walk, the sky was clear and blue, and it was jacketless warm, so suddenly spring.

He traveled one of his favorite boyhood routes: a journey he had loved during a lost time, when the growing city was less congested and the paths that wound through the riverbanks toward the tracks were much wilder. He led Michael, four, and Sara, seven, down side roads and steep, rocky banks. Michael ran out ahead. Sara preferred to stay close to her grandfather's side, holding his huge wrinkled hand as she skipped along.

Fred began the final hour of his full life with the thrill of bursting springtime freshly activated. The scent of the coming lilacs must have dulled his senses to the danger.

Then he heard the train that he did not expect. It shook the wooden ties beneath them — approaching with too much speed and momentum to stop. The conductor braked the moment he saw them, screaming with urgent blasts of his whistle.

What thunder did the quaking stir as it rippled through the nineteenth-century bridge beneath him? What form of terror did the sight and sound of the train issue to his heart? The shrill whistle started them running. Instinct must have taken over then, with Fred shouting and motioning, "Run! Run as fast as you can and don't look back — "

Fred was the president of our medical staff the day that he vanished, our congenial white-haired elder spokesman. Our staff had recently been in turmoil. Our cohesiveness was threatened by new economic realities, by the cresting waves of health care reform and managed care. Fred assumed the mantle of mediator and sounding board. He organized a series of meetings at his home — personal and informal, without minutes to record or print. This he used as a forum to try to solicit honest advice; to assimilate it, searching for the routes of pragmatic action.

Twice during that winter that preceded his untimely departure,

I had the honor to sit at his dining room table and take part in the frank discussions that he chaired.

"I think our feet will always be on solid ground whenever we *truly* put our concerns for patient care first," he told us. "I'm worried that if we don't fight for the important things *now*, that we'll be bulldozed later on." Fred's tactics leaned in favor of staking out legitimate patient care territory, and then defending it to the last ethical physician.

I sat to his left, where I could see at close range the flashes of hope and idealism as they sparked across his gray-green eyes. On the way out of one meeting, the chief of the Department of Medicine confided, "They don't make docs like ol' Fred anymore. He's a dying breed."

Recalling this months later, in the back pew at the memorial service that the hospital organized following Fred's death, I thought:

> Blessed are the Peacemakers
> For they shall see God.

My ER shift that April day had been a melee of common problems and urgent complaints. When the 3:00-to-11:00 nurses arrived, we shared a pot of fresh, strong coffee, and chattered about the glorious change in the weather. By 4:15 I had tied up loose ends and plowed through my stack of dictation. Then the paramedics went rushing by me, with their beepers blaring details of "the call," in hoarse and static tones.

For the next ten minutes I knew little more than that a nearby train had struck some people who were crossing the tracks. Then, over the radio came the information: "Medical Control . . . be advised, we have a report that there may be children involved." I recognized Marty's voice. He was one of our veteran paramedics, with fifteen years of difficult experiences under his belt, a rarely frazzled professional. Yet in the cascading inflections of his report, I heard the strident chords of *fear*.

We busied our raw nerves with practical preparation, in an atmosphere of grim silence. One of the situations we dreaded most would soon be at our doorstep. Then I heard Marty's voice again: "We're en route with a seven-year-old female, who got her foot trapped between the railroad ties."

Moments later they careened around the corner, cart wheels clanking. Marty and his partner Dick were both soaked with sweat. They took turns delivering panted bursts of further details: "Her left leg is off at the ankle. Blood pressure 120 over 80. Strong radial pulse at 100."

"She's been alert, answering every question appropriately, ever since we got t'her."

"Good breath sounds, soft abdomen. No signs of head, neck, or chest injuries."

"We had to go about twenty feet out onto the trestle to get to where she was, Doc. We found her clinging to the tracks, a few feet behind where the front wheels came to a stop."

"Her younger brother is behind us, in a second car. He doesn't have a scratch on him. The conductor told us they found him lying face-down between the tracks, under the engine."

The young girl was thin, pale. Her lips trembled. She was transferred from one cart to another by the smooth success of many hands working together. I moved up close to her right side. She stared up at me with glassy blue eyes.

"I'm the emergency room doctor. What's your name?"

"Sara." She answered in a soft voice. I stood there swaying, held by the dazed and pleading grip of her frightened eyes.

"How old are you, Sara?"

"Seven."

"Where do you hurt?"

"Just my leg."

"What happened to you?" (Her bright, steady eye contact and her clear voice and her normal vital signs began to reassure me about her airway and mental status and about the absence of life-threatening injuries.)

"I got my foot caught when we were running from the train. Grandpa tried to get it unstuck. But the train hit him, and he fell into the river."

Marty added, "One of the officers at the scene said her grandfather's a doctor on staff here."

Phil, our trauma surgeon, arrived shortly after that. I summarized what I knew as he pushed his hands into sterile gloves and approached the patient. Within seconds of focusing his eyes on her young face, he recognized the friend of his own daughter. "Sara? Sara, is that you?"

He wanted her to tell him *no*. His voice crackled — that of a father, wanting to reach out and take a suffering child in his arms.

Phil pressed on her neck, rib cage, and abdomen; then turned away. "I can't look at the leg," he said as he shuffled head down out of the trauma room. I followed him down the hall to the break room, where I poured two cups of black coffee into small Styrofoam cups. We slumped low into plastic chairs. "She slept over at our house a few weeks ago," he told me. "Call the orthopedist for me, huh? There's no way I can be objective."

When I told him that her grandfather had been with them and knocked off the trestle into the river, Phil drew in a deep breath and murmured, " 'Grandpa' must be Fred."

I placed a call to the orthopedist. I also phoned my partner, caught him just getting out of the shower. I told him what had happened, and he relieved me of duty shortly after that, starting his night shift an hour early.

Sensing the impact of the blow, the paramedics, policemen, and nurses all kept their distance from the darkened break room. Only the soft white squares of light from the viewbox on the wall illuminated, in shadow, the small circular table where Phil and I sat together — churning in the same stunned-speechless fog of disbelief.

We sipped our coffee. And stammered afterthoughts — groping for some explanation that would *undo* what we realized had happened. The wounded part longed for a healing touch. We struggled toward restored equilibrium, wanting a recaptured sense of *Order* on solid ground.

They scheduled a debriefing for the following morning. The meeting was meant to provide a forum for ventilation and helpful advice, for those of us who had caught the flak of Ground Zero. In a circle of folding chairs under the white tiles and fluorescent lights of a hospital conference room, Phil sat at three o'clock and I at seven. Scanning the circle I saw three of our best ER nurses; the policemen who handled the scene; the detective who notified the immediate family; Marty and Dick, looking haggard and pale, wearing the blank masks of the shell-shocked; and Louise, our social worker, and Father Justin, our chaplain — who between them had spent twelve hours in close quarters with the grieving family. And seated just to my left was the engineer who had been driving the train.

He had spent a sleepless night in a motel room forty miles away — driven from his own home by the anguish of a series of insensitive "prank" phone calls. This dark avenue of communication had been opened when the local news channel mentioned his name.

Talk traveled around the circle, clockwise. We first told who we were and what part we had played in "the critical incident." Then on the second swing around the circle, we shared what we remembered thinking and doing. The third circle of comments concentrated on *how it felt.*

Blood on the Tracks

One nurse cried out from the high-pitched strings of her broken heart: "What bothers me most about all this, is that such a good man had to die in such a foolish way!"

Phil poured his own words into the vacuum caused by the bleating of her pain. "I can't judge Fred. I just can't. I keep remembering all the dangerous and stupid things I did as a kid — playing chicken on my bike with oncoming trains; almost drowning trying to swim across a river; falling from a tree when I'd climbed too high. So I keep asking myself, 'Why Fred? Why him and not me?' "

The engineer was the only real eyewitness present. He was grimly silent at first, muttering only his name and cursing the insensitivity of the media and the cruelty of people. "How'd you like to pick up the phone and hear some punk askin' you, 'What's it feel like to kill a grandpa and run over a child?' "

For the better part of the first hour of our bonding discussion, he sat listening, lolling over our comments with glassy, red eyes. A world-weary weight blanched the color from his drawn expression. Then he blurted out: "I never knew Doc myself, y'know. But I heard good things about him, what he did for other people, that he was a kind man 'n all. That makes it worse for me — to have played a part in how he died."

His voice cracked and sputtered. The nurse at his side threw his arms around his slumped and shaking shoulders: "*You* didn't do anything wrong. You did everything in your power to try to prevent it. You're a victim of this tragedy too."

The engineer raised his head and continued. He had more to tell: "I'll always remember that look in his eyes. A wild look at first, glancing back over his shoulder as the brakes were squealing. I knew he didn't have a chance. He had no business being on those tracks. I just don't understand that part of it — how a smart man, like he must have been, never recognized the danger.

"But I saw what he did to try to save those kids, the clear

thinking of his final moments. The boy ran like a little gazelle; but the girl tripped, got her leg caught between the ties. He pulled on it, used both hands. And he motioned to the boy to lie down, even pushed his head flat, stretched out the boy's arms above his head. It all seemed to happen in slow motion. Freeze-frames.

"When he realized he wouldn't get the girl's foot loose in time, he wrapped his arms and chest around her. Tried to use his own body as a shield. Then he looked back, up into my eyes. Such an eerie sense of calm: I'll carry that look with me until the day that I die myself. No fear, no malice, no regrets. Like he was staring out his living room window at a blue sky."

He collapsed forward into his opened hands. Sobbing racked his bent body. Phil said, "Fred would have understood. He was a man who knew about compassion. He would not have wanted innocent people like yourself to suffer needlessly."

The engineer's outpouring of memory and feeling served as a catalyst for what the rest of the circle had kept stored up inside. It flowed and flowed, freely, until it had run its course.

"Thanks for sharing what you did," I told the engineer. "I know it must have been difficult. But I knew Fred, personally. And what you said helps me a great deal.

"I find it comforting to know that, at the end, in the midst of his crisis, Fred was thinking clearly. And that his final action . . . was *an Act of Love*."

THE GATEKEEPER

BY *Keith Ablow, M.D.*

t was shortly after one A.M. My beeper had woken me after twenty minutes of sleep. My eyes felt pasty, and my throat was dry. It took me a minute or more to gather the will to get off the cot and start down the short corridor that connected my on-call room with the emergency room. Steam pipes on either side of my head hissed as I walked by.

Etta, the emergency room triage nurse, smiled at me as I walked up to her desk. She had sat there every night for the past nineteen years. She knew how everything worked — and didn't work. "We wouldn't want you to get too far into a dream or anything," she said, without looking up. She finished gathering several sheets of paper off her desk and stapled them together. "Otherwise, you might start thinking of this place as a nightmare." She handed the sheets to me.

"Too late," I said. I looked down at the identifying information on the patient I had been summoned to evaluate. After hundreds of nights on call, I could usually tell within a sentence whether I would be spending hours to search for an open hospital bed or just minutes filling a prescription. Violence and substance abuse were bad signs; they usually meant the patient was unable to care for himself or a danger to others. A history of many hospital admissions was another ominous predictor. I had to concentrate to get my eyes to focus:

> Karl Amory. 56-year-old, divorced, homeless man complaining of depression; history of alcohol dependence, no apparent suicidal or homicidal impulses.

The negatives surprised me a bit. Many homeless patients who know the hospital system and need a place to sleep have learned to claim emphatically that they are feeling suicidal or homicidal. Hospital beds are at such a premium that any psychiatric problem short of life and death usually is made to wait until normal business hours.

Against a constant flow of would-be inpatients, one of my roles as a psychiatrist in the emergency room is that of gatekeeper, evaluating the veracity of suicidal or homicidal threats, attempting to defuse empty threats in order to justify keeping the ward census at a reasonable number.

The problems of overcrowding and understaffing are real. Very sick patients often bunk up to five in a room; some sleep in conference rooms. Many of us have been assaulted by patients in the past, and we know the ward will get too "hot" when the number of patients gets too high.

After nights when I have not admitted any patients, I have been congratulated by colleagues, slapped on the back, and affectionately called a "wall."

"What's he in the emergency room for?" I asked Etta.

"His analyst must be on vacation on the Cape," she deadpanned.

I started over to the psychiatric evaluation room. I could see my patient through the chicken-wire reinforced glass of the observation window. He was gaunt, with hollow eyes and a three-day growth of beard.

The Gatekeeper

I opened the door. The odor of alcohol mixed with sweat and urine off his layers of clothing blanketed me. I felt angry, put upon by someone who had *chosen* to drink. But only for a moment. Then I paused and reminded myself that free will is mostly an illusion. The right amount of pain at the wrong time would drive most anyone over the edge. "Mr. Amory, I'm Dr. Ablow," I said. "Would it be all right if I take a seat so we can talk for a while?"

He shrugged. "I got more time than I need."

Within ten minutes I learned that the man was a newcomer to the emergency room. He had only recently lost his job, then his wife, then his home. For a month he had wandered, drinking to forget, sleeping in shelters. Tonight he had sobered up too late to secure a shelter bed, and, alone in the freezing wind, he felt his grief and exhaustion weighing more heavily than ever.

"I need to be in the hospital," he told me. "I have to get a handle on myself."

I listened at length to his description of the losses he had suffered. "Have things gotten so bad for you that you've thought of hurting yourself?" I asked. Part of me hoped he would answer yes so that I could offer him a warm bed.

"I would never do that," he replied.

"Some people get so angry that they start thinking of hurting someone else," I hinted. "Then there's no alternative other than hospitalization."

"Look, Doc," he said. "I'm worn out. Period. I'm not mad at anyone but myself."

He denied symptoms of clinical depression or any other major mental illness. His intellect and memory were normal. He had never been admitted to a psychiatric hospital and took no medication for emotional problems. As if to offer something to reward my search for symptoms, he showed me his feet, skinned and bloody from walking the streets.

"There's no question you need help with the problems you've

talked about," I said. "I can help you follow up with the outpatient clinic downtown."

He took the slip of paper on which I had written the clinic's address and phone number. "I don't need to be in the hospital?" he asked plaintively.

"No," I said. "But I'd like to be sure you'll make an appointment with the clinic. They may decide to schedule an admission in the future."

"I will," he nodded. He looked at me expectantly. "Where do I go now?"

Just then my beeper alerted me to a phone call from outside the hospital. I excused myself and headed for the nurses' station.

In addition to performing face-to-face evaluations, being on call also means taking phone calls that come in to the hospital's main switchboard from anyone with after-hours concerns related to Psychiatry. These range from simple questions about medication side effects to pleas for help to resist suicidal or homicidal impulses. Sometimes I have had to send the police to the caller's address to bring him or her to the emergency room for evaluation.

I picked up the phone. "Hello? Dr. Ablow, psychiatry."

"I feel like jumping out of my skin," said a male voice.

"Can you tell me a little bit more about how you're feeling?" I asked.

"I'm not coming in there. You'll admit me."

"I'd really just like to know how you're — " I began. I heard the line go dead. I hung up, wondering whether the man would eventually arrive at the emergency room. Part of me hoped he would come for help, another part of me worried about getting backed up with patients. I was working a full day starting at seven A.M. and I wanted at least an hour's sleep.

Where do I go now? The words came to me again as I started back for the psychiatric evaluation room where Mr. Amory was waiting. Sometimes the answer to a question like his is simple, but I had a feeling it wouldn't be this time. I knew none of the local shelters had any beds left, but I called and checked anyhow. No luck. I called the admitting office of the hospital and found out they had already used up the few beds available to "board" patients who didn't qualify for admission.

I turned around and headed out the emergency room doors. The security guard was standing at the entrance, leaning against the brick wall, like he usually did. "Harry," I said. "I got a homeless man back there who got to the shelter too late to get in. He's not suicidal or homicidal, so I can't admit him. Can he sleep in the lobby?"

Harry rolled his eyes. He is a big man, with a big heart, but he needs his job. "You know the answer to that question."

"I know. It's against the rules. But what difference — "

"I agree with you. Call the CEO at home, why don't you?"

I rubbed my eyes. "Where, then?"

"What about the airport? They let 'em sleep on the floor there, sometimes."

"Are the buses still running?"

"No."

I stopped by Etta's desk to ask whether the hospital petty cash fund might have ten dollars for a cab to the airport.

"Used up," she said. "Last of it went before nine."

I dragged myself back to Amory. "I can't find a place anywhere for you," I said, shaking my head.

"It's cold," he said. "It'll be four, five hours before it's light."

Etta opened the door. I excused myself and stepped outside. "You've got another patient," she said. "He's a graduate student. Crying uncontrollably. He says he wants to die."

"Put him in Room Two and make sure someone watches him until I can get to him," I said. "I'll be done here in a few minutes."

I walked back to Amory's room and sat down. I reached into the pocket of my scrubs and handed him three dollar bills. "I'd hop on the subway to the airport," I said.

He started putting his socks over the medicated gauze a nurse had wrapped around his injured feet. "The subway's dangerous," he said.

I stood up. "I wouldn't want to ride it myself, but there's not a lot more I can do."

That was a lie, of course, and I believe we both knew it. I'd only part with three dollars for a person in no immediate danger with nowhere to go.

The two twenties upstairs in my call room — enough for a taxi and a motel — stayed there. My car, good shelter from the wind, was parked right out front. I didn't even think of unlocking it for him. I have family and friends who live not thirty minutes from the hospital, with extra beds. I wouldn't think of asking them to open their homes to a stranger. And as a psychiatrist, empathy is my calling.

Why wouldn't I do more? The reason is that I had hit my internal "wall." Part of it was fear. I have learned that I really don't know much about anyone after an hour together.

Moreover, despite all my attempts to banish it, I still harbor the prejudice that those who cannot sustain themselves in society are less likely to be bound by society's rules. Losing all one's possessions raises the suspicion that a person is somehow out of control in every way.

I felt — unfairly or not — that to get involved with this patient would put me at risk of being physically harmed or at least exploited. Maybe I was afraid of being overwhelmed, that if I truly extended myself to one homeless man, what would prevent my being used up by the sheer bulk of homeless people?

As a child, I was more than once admonished by a teacher not to share candy with a friend if I didn't have enough for everyone. So I kept it to myself.

I believe I also had myself convinced that my restraint had a therapeutic component. Perhaps, I thought, this man had not yet fallen far enough to take hold of himself, to stop drinking, to get another job. And even if he didn't spend the money on booze, a room tonight might be no more than a bandage obscuring an infected sore, allowing whatever infection was at work to do more lasting damage. What, indeed, if his disorder was a dependent personality? I would be playing into his pathological inability to be self-sufficient.

The problem is that these are theories.

I know that there are many people who need to be taken care of. But at two A.M., the job of distinguishing those who need firm limits from those who need warm beds from those who need to be left alone was overwhelming.

So, headed for Room 2, I was left with the nagging guilt that I could, or should, have done more for Karl Amory. He was not the first patient I worried I had let down. And I knew he would not be the last.

HALLOWEEN

BY *Robert Marion, M.D.*

I was on call last night in the pediatric emergency room and I learned an important lesson: If you want to come across as compassionate and empathetic, if you want people to trust you and have faith in your judgment, it's probably not a good idea to go to work dressed like Bozo the Clown. I know that because I did go to work dressed like Bozo the Clown yesterday and things didn't go all that well. In fact, it was one of the worst nights of my life.

I guess I should explain. Yesterday was October 31, Halloween. The day before, our on-call team had talked it over and we all decided that, since we were pediatricians and since Halloween was such an important holiday for kids, we should get into the spirit by coming to work in costume. To be honest, it didn't seem like such a good idea to me, but as one of the interns on the team, I couldn't exactly tell my senior resident, "No, I think that's stupid, I think wearing a costume all day in the emergency room is a dumb idea." So after I finished work on Friday night, I went home and tried to find my Bozo costume.

I knew it had to be around somewhere. I'd had the costume since my first year of medical school; it had been given to me by one of my classmates who had found it buried in his closet during a housecleaning frenzy that had occurred while studying for our neuroscience final. The costume consisted of a wild, orange wig, a glue-on bulbous nose, a multicolored polyester smock, and big, floppy clown shoes; it also came complete with a makeup kit. My classmate was going to discard it; I figured it might someday come in handy, so I took it and proceeded to lose it in my own closet.

After searching for about a half hour, I finally found the thing, still in its original box, squashed into a back corner of that closet. I took it out and put on the smock, shoes, and wig: They still looked good as new. Early Saturday morning, I put on the costume again, applied the makeup carefully, following the instructions on the back of the box, and peered into the mirror: I have to admit, I looked pretty goofy. But I guess that's the look I was trying to achieve: I could have been a clone of the famous television clown.

I may have looked goofy, but when I reached the hospital, I quickly discovered that compared with some of my colleagues, I looked as conservative as a Wall Street banker. Peter Carson, our senior resident, who's about six feet three and weighs at least 250 pounds, was dressed as a ballerina, in a tutu, leotard, and size thirteen toe shoes. Terry Tanner, one of the junior residents, came dressed as the pope; she spent the entire evening blessing people and inviting them to kiss her ring. And two of my fellow interns came dressed as killer bees, wearing yellow-and-black body suits, long antennae, and long, thin stingers that looked like sitting down was going to be kind of a challenge. Even Lucille Turner, the emergency room's crabby head nurse, made an effort, but frankly, her costume wasn't much of a stretch: She came dressed as the Wicked Witch of the West. All in all, we presented quite a tableau to the infirm and downtrodden of the Bronx.

Well, at least the kids seemed to like it. They all looked kind of stunned when they first came in from the waiting room and saw us. But, almost immediately, each began to smile, and pretty quickly the smiles turned into laughs. We had bowls of candy spread around the place, and the kids were helping themselves (at least the ones who hadn't come in with gastroenteritis). Most of the parents seemed skeptical: It's one thing to go to the emergency room after you've been kept awake all night by a screaming three-year-old to be seen by a competent, or at least a semicompetent, doctor. It's quite another, however, to have to go through that and then wait an hour or so and finally get called in to find out your kid's going to be seen by Bozo the Clown. But I think at least most people left thinking that it was a good idea and weren't we a nice group of doctors to think of the kids.

The day was going pretty well; I was even beginning to think that I'd been wrong, that maybe this really was a good idea. That's when we got the phone call.

It was about nine o'clock, right in the middle of the busiest time of the evening. We got a call from EMS, saying that they were bringing in a traumatic arrest. So Bozo the Clown, the six-foot-three-inch prima ballerina, the Wicked Witch of the West, the pope, and one of the killer bees each left the patient with whom he or she had been working and, in nervous anticipation, crowded into the trauma area.

After about two minutes, we heard a commotion coming from the adult emergency room. The emergency medical technicians were running down the ER's corridor, pushing a stretcher. One of the techs was on the side, performing chest compressions, while the other was at the back, working the ambu bag. With them hovering over the patient, it was hard to see at first who the patient actually was.

It turned out to be an eight-year-old boy. He had been out trick-or-treating, and, after stepping out into the street between two parked cars, he'd been nailed by a passing van. The driver of the van panicked when he realized what had happened and, not knowing what to do, he'd slammed the gears into reverse, running the boy over a second time.

Someone called 911, and the ambulance got to the scene within ten minutes. They started CPR out on the street, but you could tell it wasn't doing the boy much good. He was pulseless and apneic, and when they hooked him up to a monitor, he was flat-line. He was clearly DOA.

We knew it would probably prove to be useless, but we did everything anyway. Peter Carson intubated him, Terry Tanner started pumping his chest, and Bruce Davidson (one of the killer bees) and I tried to get lines in. I somehow got one in his right arm, which was a miracle in itself, and we started pushing bicarb and epi, but nothing helped.

At about that point the trauma surgeons came in and said they wanted to crack the kid's chest. None of us believed it would help, but we figured we had to give this boy every possible chance to survive; besides, when three surgeons walk up to you with scalpels in their hands and say they'd like to crack a patient's chest, it's hard to say no.

It took no more than two minutes to get the boy's chest exposed and when it was, it became clear that the code was over: we found that he had a bronchopleural fistula. The impact of the van had caused the left main stem bronchus, the main windpipe to the left lung, to tear in half; the oxygen that we were forcing into the boy's windpipe through the endotracheal tube was ending up in the pleural space outside the lung, causing an ever-worsening tension pneumothorax.

I walked out of the trauma area, and the boy's mother was standing there less than ten feet away. She was literally being held up by one of the emergency room nurses. She said, "Doctor, how is he? Is he going to be okay?" I didn't see any way out; I was too upset to come up with a lie. So that's when I, dressed in my Bozo wig, my Bozo makeup, my Bozo shoes, and my Bozo smock, which was now soaked through with her son's blood, told that woman that her boy had died.

ROBERT MARION, M.D.

She went crazy. She started crying and fell down on the floor. I felt like a total idiot standing there dressed like that, and there was nothing, absolutely nothing, I could do to change anything. One of the hospital administrators appeared and he, the nurse, and I managed to lift the mother up off the floor. The administrator then led the crying woman out of the ER.

I left the emergency room, too; I just couldn't see another patient just then, not looking the way I did. Taking the stairs two at a time, I ran up to the operating room's locker room, quiet and deserted at that hour. In the silence, I scrubbed the stupid makeup off my face; I then took off the costume and replaced it with a fresh set of scrubs. Before leaving the locker room to return to the ER, I bundled up the wig, shoes, and smock and threw the whole bloody mess into the trash.

I don't think I'll ever dress up in a clown suit again; I'm afraid the memories of that dead little boy and his mother will be permanently entwined with the costume. And next year, if I'm on call on Halloween again, I don't think I'm going to dress up.

STUDENT DOCTOR

BY *Mickey Zucker Reichert, M.D.*

The steel and whitewash of Savenberg's emergency room formed a startling contrast to the lecture hall and laboratories that had filled Jennifer Klein's first two years of medical school. The bleeps of cardiac monitors, the bump and scrape of gurney wheels, and the shouts of medical personnel formed a numbing, indecipherable cacophony. Occasionally, the paramedics' call radio spewed static into the tumult. Nothing had prepared her for the myriad clashing odors: the salt smell of blood and the acid stench of vomit mingled with cloying cleaning solutions and alcohol. The reek of rotting flesh pervaded the hallways from the patient moaning in Room 6. Klein's stomach lurched as she whisked down the corridor in Bob Peterson's wake, her short, white coat flapping behind her, tuning forks, stethoscope, and portable oto/ophthalmoscope jangling in her pockets.

A third-year resident, Peterson had become Klein's lifeline in a world she had chosen but now seemed ill suited to survive. Two years of daily classes on anatomy, physiology, and pathology, a year of dissecting a cadaver and studying minutiae under a microscope had taxed her mind to its limit. She had scored As, yet now those seemed a sham. The reality of the ER bore no relationship she could fathom to the words and concepts she returned, verbatim, to the professors on their tests. She felt incapable of reconciling her studies to actual patients.

Sweat beaded Klein's forehead, and her palms went suddenly clammy. She flicked back her short, dark locks with restless strokes, surreptitiously wiping away the perspiration. Her fingers seemed awkward, disconnected from her nervous system; and panic accompanied a thought that seemed to spring from nowhere: Something about her mind did not function properly, making it unable to translate book learning into practicality. She had done well in school only because her brain handled paperwork competently. Soon, the truth would emerge, and the world would know that Jennifer Klein had no diagnostic or treatment acumen.

Peterson whirled abruptly. Only Klein's instinctive side step saved them from a collision. She studied the resident's round, gentle features. His dark eyes seemed cowlike, clashing with a stance that radiated confidence. His slender form, almost too skinny, stood spare inches taller than her five-foot eight-inch frame; and she believed she might outweigh him. He wore a dress shirt, pants, and a colorful tie tucked through the buttonholes. Unlike her in her white coat, stuffed full of necessary supplies, he carried only a stethoscope around his neck and a penlight in his breast pocket. "You're nervous, aren't you, Jennifer?"

"Um . . . yes," Klein admitted, daunted despite the kindness he had thus far shown her. "How can you tell?"

Peterson smiled. "Well, in addition to the fact that it's the first day of your first rotation and everybody's nervous then . . ."

Klein managed a thin-lipped smile.

". . . you just followed me into the men's room."

"Oh, my God." Without allowing herself a glance to confirm Peterson's words, Klein flinched, turned, and fled. She ran without thought or direction. Her cheeks felt on fire, and she mentally berated her stupidity. She had now demonstrated her inadequacy

Student Doctor

to the one person in Savenberg's ER who had not thoroughly intimidated her.

Klein's headlong flight sent her crashing into a willowy surgeon. Pain slammed her face and neck, and momentum flung her to the floor. Papers spiraled in every direction, followed by the thunk of a chart.

Klein twisted her head to assess the damage. The surgeon had pitched to one knee, and his face darkened from scarlet to nearly purple. Klein watched in helpless horror as the last few papers he had carried fluttered to the ground. He opened his mouth, but no words emerged. Instead, he pinned her with a glare of withering disdain that made her wish she were small enough to hide under the materials cart. "I'm sorry," she squeaked.

Rising, the surgeon loosed a wordless noise of disgust. His name tag identified him as J. Kevin Hartwell, M.D. Without acknowledging her apology, he gestured at the scattered papers and the partially emptied chart. "Handle it. With more grace than you've demonstrated so far." He hurried off, clearly too busy to deal with the mess Klein had caused.

Stupid, stupid, stupid . . . Klein's mind shifted into a cyclic cadence as she carefully shuffled the papers into a pile on top of the chart. Nurses, orderlies, and doctors stepped carefully around her as she worked. *Stupid, stupid.* Klein carried the stack to a table, hooking a chair with one foot and plopping into the seat with a self-deprecating sigh. *Stupid.*

An elderly nurse turned Klein a shy smile and a wink. "Why don't you let me handle that?"

The idea of putting another person out for her clumsiness appalled Klein. "Oh. No, thank you. It was my mistake."

"I insist. You've got more important things to do." The nurse slid the chart from Klein's grip and dragged it in front of herself. Though the nurse spoke amiably, Klein thought she detected a hint of condescension. The nurse did not trust her to replace the papers in proper order, and with good cause. Klein had never before looked in a patient's chart.

"Thank you," Klein said in a shrill whisper, wishing her normal voice would return. Her throat felt pinched.

One set of footsteps sorted themselves from a cluster, deliberately headed toward Klein. She turned to face Bob Peterson. The resident gave her an encouraging smile. "Ah, there you are," he said as if he had completely forgotten the circumstances of their separation. He ran a hand through his mop of straw-colored hair, jumbling it into spiky patches. "We've got a patient in the trauma room."

Klein leapt to her feet, determined to present a better side of herself than she had thus far shown the ER staff. "I'm ready," she stated, feeling anything but. She followed Peterson toward Room 1.

The resident presented the case as they walked: "Forty-six-year-old black female who slipped on a country driveway. Got about a six-centimeter laceration on the posterior right calf. No other injuries."

"Sutures?" Klein appreciated the straightforward case.

"Yeah. But first I'll need to explore the wound. Make sure there's no gravel or other foreign bodies in there."

Klein nodded her agreement, wanting to kick herself for not considering such an obvious need. Once Peterson mentioned it, it seemed painfully apparent.

Peterson entered the trauma room, brushing aside a striped curtain that hid the patient from view. It parted to reveal a middle-aged, heavyset woman seated on the standard wheeled table, locked in place. A sleek, patterned dress fell just past her knees. Torn pantyhose hung from the back of the room's only chair, and a pair of dress shoes peeked neatly from beneath it. She clutched a square of bloody gauze to the back of her right foreleg. A metal tray held a bundle wrapped in a green towel with a package of size 8 gloves thrown casually atop it. A plastic bottle of saline, a 3-cc syringe with attached needle still in its wrapper, three iodine wipes, and a bottle of lidocaine lay beside the other objects.

"All right, Ms. Harmon. This is student doctor Klein. She's going to watch me work, if you don't mind." Peterson jerked the curtain closed without awaiting a reply.

Klein marveled at how Peterson had presented the situation. His tone implied that objecting would make Harmon an odd and irascible patient without sounding at all offensive.

Harmon gave Klein a smile. "So you're learning how to sew me up?"

Klein returned a shy grin. "Yes, ma'am."

"Roll over, please, Ms. Harmon." Peterson dragged over a portable lamp that Klein had not previously noticed, while the woman rearranged herself prone on the table. Peterson adjusted the flexible neck and tapped the switch. Light bathed Harmon's skin, revealing white lines of dryness forming irregular scales and a gash clotted with dried blood.

Peterson waved Klein to his side. Opening a drawer in the equipment cart located in every room, he removed a pair of non-sterile gloves. After prepping the wound with iodine, he opened the green cloth, exposing multiple instruments, needles, syringes, and a metal bowl. He removed his gloves. He opened the needle package but did not remove the paper, then flipped the lid from the lidocaine. Without touching needle or syringe, he drew up 2 cc of medication and dumped the syringe amid the sterile instruments. Twisting the cap from the saline, he poured a generous amount into the bowl. Turning his attention to the gloves, he peeled the wrapper completely open. He wiggled his right hand partway into one glove, slid his awkwardly gloved fingers under the cuff of the other, and flicked it over his left. Rearranging each finger into its proper hole with a snap of rubber, he clasped his palms together.

Klein watched every step with fanatical interest. She had never seen a sterile procedure performed and wanted to capture every nuance of the process.

Peterson hefted the lidocaine-filled syringe and screwed on a 25-gauge needle, the smallest the emergency room stocked. "All right, Ms. Harmon. There'll be a small stick and burn. After that, you shouldn't feel any pain."

Harmon nodded, then folded her arms like a pillow beneath her head. The location of the injury did not allow her to oversee Peterson's work, which did not seem to bother her. She looked peaceful, comfortable, her faith in Peterson deriving from his calm self-assurance. A study in opposites, Klein felt fidgety as a child trapped listening to a boring, seven-hour sermon. As closely as she watched, she found it difficult to recall every step in order. She stared as Peterson inserted the needle at the wound's edge, drew back, then pressed the plunger, creating a weal at the site. "That's the worst of it." He continued injecting around the wound, advancing and withdrawing the needle in a slow pattern. As he worked, he chatted with the patient, about her life and the details of the accident. Focused on his technique, Klein let the conversation slip past her, mostly unheard.

Using the sterile instruments, Peterson probed the wound, never ceasing his discourse with the patient about unrelated matters. His ministrations revealed the depth of the laceration, well into the muscle tissue. His inspection restarted the bleeding, and a bright red trickle wound toward the patient's ankle. Acid churned in the pit of Klein's stomach, and she glanced at the tray table to avoid looking at the wound. *Oh, my God, I'm squeamish!* The realization surprised as well as horrified her. She recalled how easy cutting into the cadaver had seemed, the bloodless, preserved flesh yielding easily to the knife. The minor cuts, bruises, and scrapes she had accumulated over the years never bothered her; but the image of Peterson's hemostat gouging into Harmon's laceration, scarlet rivulets trailing, proved too much.

More afraid of humiliating herself by fainting than of missing the process, Klein allowed herself only occasional glimpses of the lavage and suturing. Terror stole over her. *All those years of medical school. The endless nights of studying. Tens of thousands in loans. And I can't stand the sight of blood.* She hiccuped, fighting tears. *I'll never be a doctor.* Moisture blurred her vision, and it took an effort of will to keep herself from sobbing. All the compassion, all the desire to help humanity meant nothing if she swooned every time a patient bled.

"All finished," Peterson announced at length. "Nothing left but the cleanup."

Klein wiped her eyes with the back of her hand, watching the resident smear antibacterial salve over the neat row of knots, then apply a cover of gauze and tape.

"I'll be right back with the paperwork." Peterson trundled out the door with Klein directly on his heels. The hallway air seemed fresh after the confines of Room 1, and the strange combination of cleaners and medicines reawakened her nausea. She watched as Peterson took a double sheet of instructions from a pile, stamped it with the patient's ID plate, then scrawled his signature onto a line. "Now I just have her sign it, give her her copy, and we're done." He glanced at the clock, then at the white board listing rooms and patients. "It's quiet enough. We can go to lunch."

Lunch? Klein jerked her eyes to the clock, which read 11:50 A.M. After orientation, she had seen only two patients: Ms. Harmon and a vomiting, dehydrated infant. Klein had felt certain the baby boy suffered from gastroenteritis, but Peterson had made the correct diagnosis of pyloric stenosis with an ease that seemed impossible to master. He had palpated an olive-sized mass near the liver that Klein could scarcely locate, by touch and imagination, even after he placed her fingers directly on it. The process floored her, the conversion from textbook description to reality a talent that seemed so natural to others but that her brain, apparently, lacked. Every doctor, from the residents to the ER attendings to the specialists, seemed so capable and poised while she bumbled and stumbled like a toddler learning to walk. Logically, she knew their ability stemmed from experience, but she could not help secretly fearing that she would never understand their skills. If only patients came with diagnoses tattooed to their foreheads.

Klein looked into Bob Peterson's eyes and found a camaraderie there that she desperately needed. It seemed foolish and dangerous to confess her weakness to anyone, especially a resident who might evaluate her abilities as a doctor and partially determine whether or not she graduated. But, right now, she needed solace more. "How could you do that?"

Peterson blinked. "Lunch?"

"No, the suturing."

Peterson misunderstood the question, perhaps deliberately. "It's not as hard as it looks. I'll teach you the stitch."

Before Klein could correct his misconception, he steered her toward the supply cart. "Grab some suture, a needle holder, and scissors. I'll show you over lunch." He shook the papers for Ms. Harmon. "Be back in a minute."

"Right." Klein bellied up to the supply cart, inadequacies forgotten for the moment. The quiet routine of searching for the required objects restored her composure, and she was glad she had not confessed her qualms to her preceptor resident. Even Bob Peterson probably had few suggestions for a weak-willed medical student except to bully through the discomfort and get on with her training. Klein scanned the labels on the supply cart's drawers, pulling out a small scissors and a needle holder. She headed for the varied suture materials, seeking one in the same color package as Peterson had used.

Klein had just separated one from the box when J. Kevin Hartwell glided up beside her. Snatching the package from her hand, he read the label. "Wouldn't sew a dog with that crap." He flung it back into the box, selected the variety he needed, and headed away without another word.

Klein's heart beat a rapid, startled cadence, and she waited until it normalized before selecting another package of suture. She doubted the material or size of it mattered during a teaching session, and she promised herself to avoid dealing with the surgeon, if at all possible, in the future. A month of working around that man would surely spark nightmares.

Peterson returned shortly after Hartwell disappeared. "Ready?"

"Ready," Klein returned halfheartedly. Learning would serve her little good without the nerve to apply her lesson.

Peterson's ER attending, Dr. Averell Javin, met resident and student at the white board after lunch. He kept his thinning salt-and-pepper hair combed in long strands over his bald spot and sported a neat, gray beard that softened his jowly face. "There's a chest pain in Room Seven." He directed Peterson. "I'll handle the OB case in twelve."

Peterson darted off in the indicated direction. Klein started to follow, but Javin seized her arm. "You're working with us, right?"

"Yes, sir," Klein said, desperately trying to steady her voice. The broad giant of a man daunted her worse than the rude surgeon she had vowed to avoid. This one held the future of her career in his hands.

"Great. I need you to suture in the trauma room." Javin inclined his head toward Room 1, then bustled off toward Room 12 without further instructions.

Klein froze, torn between chasing after Peterson or calling to Javin that he had sorely misinterpreted the level of her experience. If she dawdled long enough, Peterson would finish with his patient and assist her.

Klein sucked air through her teeth, a new emotion fluttering in her chest, a faint, unrecognizable spark. It strengthened gradually even as a million doubts raced through her mind, paralyzing her. *You've seen it done. You know the stitch.* Under Peterson's tutelage, she had practiced the knots over sandwiches, using a napkin as their patient. The idea of attempting such a thing seemed madness, yet even the most eminent cardiac surgeon once faced a first challenge. *What if I faint during the procedure? What if I contaminate the patient?* Klein forced the negatives aside. Her future as a physician depended upon pleasing her attending. Surely, he had grown accustomed to directing residents and more seasoned students, not realizing it was Klein's first day out of a classroom.

Klein headed for the trauma room, drawing images of Peterson back to the foreground, wishing she had watched the whole procedure on Ms. Harmon from beginning to end. The curtain was open, revealing a slender, wizened man in a stained T-shirt and patched jeans. The odor of beer wafted from him. A red-headed, male nurse dabbed at his scalp with alcohol and a gauze pad, and the metal tray held its assortment of necessities, lacking only a pair of sterile gloves. Klein appreciated that the nurse had handled the materials. Left to her own devices, she would surely have forgotten something.

"Hold still please, Mr. Weathers." The nurse held direct pressure on the gauze with a gloved hand. "Good afternoon, Dr. Klein."

Klein resisted the urge to look behind her, unused to a title that did not yet legally belong to her. Nevertheless, she did not correct the nurse. Adding the word "student" would only frighten the patient, and she could scarcely stand the additional problems that might create.

"Mr. Weathers had a little too much to drink. He thinks he cut his head getting out of his car, but he's not sure. He didn't feel anything, just noticed the blood."

"Hello, Mr. Weathers," Klein managed.

"Hello, Doctor," he returned.

"Here, hold this." The nurse took the patient's hand and placed it on top of the gauze pad. "Don't let go."

Weathers obeyed, and the nurse slipped around to assist Klein. "What size gloves do you take?"

Klein had no idea. "Um . . . ," she started, then stopped. Peterson, she recalled, used eights, and her hands were smaller. "Seven," she tried.

Dutifully, the nurse pulled a pair of size 7 from the drawer. "Is there anything else you need?"

About a year's worth of experience. Klein kept the thought to herself. "No. Thank you. I can handle it from here." She only hoped saying it would make it true.

With a nod, the nurse headed from the room, pulling the curtain closed behind her.

Jennifer Klein's heart pounded a meteoric cadence, and she focused on her breathing to keep from hyperventilating. She ignored the patient, concentrating on duplicating every step of Peterson's procedure. To miss one raised the possibility of contaminating her sterile field, and the patient. At the least, she would require a second prepping and gloving.

Klein completed the initial steps with a methodical slowness, checking and double-checking every action. At length, she had the scalp prepped, the lidocaine drawn, and all materials in place. The gloves seemed to take a century to align, fingers refusing to find their proper places. Finally, she finished the process, only to realize she had forgotten the work lamp. She studied the wound, a flap with two straight edges. She could not bear to start over now. The overhead fluorescents would have to illuminate it well enough.

Placing the small needle on the syringe of lidocaine, Klein stared at it a moment. Only then, she realized she had never given a shot before. She looked at Weathers. He seemed calm, oblivious to her consternation. So long as she did not inject the lidocaine intravenously, she could not harm him. Even a layman knew to draw back on the plunger before injecting. *Calm. Calm. Calm. Calm.* Tense as a coiled spring despite her mantra, Klein jabbed the needle into the edge of the wound, forgetting to warn Weathers of the stick and burn.

Weathers did not flinch. Apparently, the beer numbed him well enough. Drawing back without a blood return, Klein injected, working her way around the wound as Peterson had done. When she reached the end, she held an empty syringe, remembering only then that Peterson had used about half as much for a similarly sized injury. *Used enough to anesthetize a mastiff,* she chastised herself. She returned the syringe to the tray. Next, she set to suturing, awkwardly tying the knots she had practiced, for the first time, at lunch.

Weathers's voice broke the long silence on the third stitch. "So Doc, what do you guys practice on anyway?"

Klein jumped, nearly gouging herself with the needle. "Excuse me?"

"What do docs practice on? Oranges? Dogs?"

The old Palmolive commercial filled Klein's mind. *You're soaking in it.* "And other things." She dodged the question, inserting the needle with a clumsy twist for the fourth and final suture. Only as she tied it did she realize she had worried so much for procedure, she had completely forgotten about the blood. Now, she could see it had slimed her gloves and dried on Weathers's scalp. Strangely, the sight no longer bothered her. Without a word, she cleaned away the dried flakes, peeled off her gloves, and applied antibiotic salve between the knots. Her judicious use of lidocaine would make the wound swell slightly more than normal, but it otherwise looked fine.

Student Doctor

Klein left the trauma room on shaky legs, uncertain whether to collapse, vomit, or dance a jig. *I did it!* Nervousness gradually gave way to an excitement that thrilled through her entire being. A smile snaked its way onto her face and would not be banished. Snatching an instructing sheet from the pile, she stamped it with Weathers's plate. Dr. Peterson sat at the main table, discussing his case with Javin.

An hour ago, Klein would have hovered quietly in the background, awaiting acknowledgment. Now, she strode directly to the resident's side, pausing only for a lull in the dialogue. "Pardon me. Would you cosign this for me?"

Peterson looked at the paper, then at Klein. A grin nearly as large as her own split his features, and he gave her a broad wink. He signed the page, then reminded gently. "He has to sign, too. When you're done, head over to X ray and look up Carol Johnson's film. That's the lady I'm seeing. I'll meet you there."

Clutching her paper like a proud parent, Klein headed back to Weathers's room.

Jennifer Klein held Carol Johnson's chest film, waiting for her turn at the lighted viewbox. At length, the pediatrics resident finished with his X ray and stepped aside for her to take his place. Before Klein could clip Johnson's X ray in place, Dr. Hartwell moved in and slapped an abdominal on the box. Startled, Klein leapt into retreat. Then, emboldened by her recent success, she examined the X ray over the surgeon's shoulder. She knew little radiology yet, but she saw no better way to learn than to ask questions. Pointing to a shadow near the stomach, she asked politely, "Excuse me, Dr. Hartwell. Could you please tell me what that is?"

Hartwell stiffened. Gradually, he looked toward Klein, as if the effort of moving his head taxed him beyond endurance. "Is it your *patient?*"

"No."

"Then why do you care?" Hartwell returned to his examination.

Klein felt as if the surgeon had taken an ax and hacked her legs out from under her. As before, she wanted to slink away, but this time she had an answer. "I care because I'm a student doctor who wants to become a competent doctor." She added before she could think to stop herself, "I could learn a lot from you, too, if you weren't so damned arrogant!"

Hartwell's eyes widened and his nostrils flared. Without further comment, he snatched his X ray down and stormed from the room.

Klein clamped her hand over her mouth, at once wishing she had never spoken and glad that she finally had. Then, she heard a sound behind her. It started softly, a gentle clapping, joined by others, growing into unmistakable applause. Klein whirled with a gasp. Until that moment, she had believed herself and Hartwell the only ones in the room. Now, she recognized Peterson and Javin among a handful of nurses and a few strangers as well.

"I-I'm sorry," Klein said, her action unforgivable.

"I'm not," Javin said gruffly. "The jerk had it coming, and there aren't many medical students who'll give it to guys like that. You're going to do fine here, Klein. I don't know how much medicine we'll teach you, but you've got time for that. Part of becoming a doctor is learning to handle people, including patronizing clods. Good start."

Klein could scarcely believe Javin's reaction. "I'm not so sure that's a good thing, sir. Making enemies my first day."

Peterson shook his head vigorously, still smiling.

Javin laughed. "Enemies? Don't be ridiculous. Men like Hartwell don't respect anyone who doesn't stand up to them. By tomorrow, he'll take you under his wing. You'll see. And you're right, there's a lot he can teach you. For all of his pomposity, he's a damn good surgeon. Now get that X ray up there, and let me teach you, too."

Klein complied, warmth filling every crevice of her being. From an alcoholic named Weathers had come the first spark of a confidence she so desperately needed. She would never forget her first patient and the lesson he taught her.

And one day, Jennifer Klein hoped, she would become a damn good surgeon, too.

THE HANDS

BY *John Stone, M.D.*

The Emergency Department is usually quiet early Saturday mornings. Things that hurt too badly have caused the owners of such pain to come in earlier — and the accidents haven't as yet had time to happen. But the early morning is a favorite time for the elephant-on-the-chest discomfort of a heart attack: it may come on during the rapid eye movement portion of sleep, that part of sleep associated with dreaming. With a thumping dream, good or bad, the eyes roll under the lids like marbles in oil. It can be as though you're running while lying down, your body tense, heart pumping wildly to no purpose, blood pressure up. Perhaps that's when it happened to him.

What we know is that he sat up on the side of the bed, still, as when he went to sleep, 39 years old. And complained of pain. An ambulance was called and got to him quickly: no question what he had or what must be done. Lying there, hurtling there under the siren, he stopped breathing. Resuscitation was begun: pump, breathe, pump, breathe. Two minutes from the hospital. Radio the Emergency Department: *Roger. Man with chest pain. Just arrested. ETA 1 minute. Get the doors open.*

Galvanized is the word for what happens then in the Emergency

Department: a flurry of white coats, hands, legs, linen. Drugs, EKG ready. The whip of the siren. *They're on the ramp.*

39, I keep thinking. *Damn!*

As the EKG machine is hooked up, the tube for breathing pure oxygen is put down. *He's pinker. Keep pumping on the chest.* Nothing on the EKG. Not a thing, just the mechanical jumps of the needle as the Resident pumps a perfect 60 times a minute. Nothing to shock. Flat line. Drugs — that's what we need: *epinephrine, bicarb. Hurry. Keep pumping!*

The resident is sweating heavily and is relieved when someone offers to take over for him. Nothing works. No drug is helping. Try another. *Try calcium.*

I swear his hand moved — no, his *arm* moved. *Both* arms are moving! His heart is still dead, but he's moving his arms! *God. Never Saw That Happen Before.*

The hands come up on his chest to the hands of the pumping Resident and *push* them away. He's making a sound around the tube in his mouth.

Check the EKG. Stop pumping. Check it.

Nothing.

The hands fall down lifeless again. Pump.

Pump! Try some more epinephrine. Nothing. Straight line. Nothing on his own.

Get me a pacemaker.

The hands come up again, pushing away the doctor's hands.

Stop pumping so I can see the EKG. Nothing. The man's hands fall down again as the pumping is interrupted momentarily. We're keeping him alive but he won't let us.

Here's the pacemaker. Keep pumping. Check the blood gases.

The pacemaker doesn't help. He has no pump left. His heart muscle is gone. We keep trying, pumping. The hands come up and fall back down. Death is fighting off life and the living.

We work for hours. The hands are weaker; they do not rise as often; they do not rise at all; they do not move. We have lost in spite of everything. The something that waits inside us all for the first falter and stumble of the heart has won.

I hope his wife is a strong spirit. I'd like to tell her about the hands. About how he struggled. How we hurt with him in that purgatory until we were all rendered innocent of everything we might have been guilty of, then and tomorrow.

THE BOX

BY *Julian Orenstein, M.D.*

S ome nights are foreshadowed by tragedy. Now, I normally do not believe that a full moon results in any more or less carnage than nights when the moon is in some lesser phase, nor do I really think that the tides of flotsam and human jetsam that come into the emergency room occur with any predictability the way many of my colleagues do when they say that "things come in threes." But on some nights there are . . . *hints*. Sometimes it is a purposeful act on my part: If I've read an article on the latest data on the usefulness — or lack thereof — of steroids in meningitis, I will see a kid with full-blown meningococcemia. Or if I've reviewed, for the tenth time, the pathologic processes involved in near-drowning episodes, damned if some poor kid doesn't come in who was just pulled out of a bathtub or a pool.

I've thought about this because most nights are so damn boring from start to finish. In my ER I work evenings and see children. Most of them have nothing worse than the current virus du jour, or trivial injuries that are no cause for concern or deep thought. I think I would go crazy if all I ever saw were these kids. I was trained exclusively in Pediatrics, but since I work in a hospital whose ER takes care of everyone, I pick up adult cases half of the time, the ones who aren't having strokes or heart attacks. If I approach them as overgrown kids with no parent to stop them from whining, I find that they're not too different from children. And while worried parents bring their children in for some pretty strange reasons, sometimes, the things that adults come into the ER with are *wild* by comparison.

On one memorable night a stripper came in with a rash that glowed in black light. The customers loved it, but she had had syphilis once before and wanted to know if she had it again. She did. The same night a woman from Kuwait strayed in who wanted a pregnancy test. She had come to America for a vacation and stayed with a friend who had promised to take care of her. If she was pregnant when she returned to Kuwait, her husband would have her executed. Her friend had indeed taken very good care of her: She was pregnant. I never knew what became of her.

Sometimes the foreshadows disappear and nothing happens. By the end of the shift, at two or so in the morning, I will have long forgotten the mist that had hung so palpably over the start of the evening. Most of the time, in fact, that is the way things go. I come in to work with a spooky feeling of dread, and then it's just the same old routine for ten or twelve hours.

All it takes to deliver on this threat, though, is two words: "line one," meaning that there is a doctor, nurse, or paramedic, *someone,* on the telephone out there somewhere, calling in to tell me that there is some kid coming my way who is dead or dying, and that I should get ready. Sue Black is usually the nurse who delivers me the worst news; I know enough to be worried when she tells me, "Pick up on line one, there's a doc sending in a sick one."

I don't like Sue, but it's not because of that. Sue, a.k.a. Cobrahead, Bearclaw, the Beast. There probably isn't a species in the animal kingdom she hasn't been compared to. Her tall head of red hair is something I can *feel* before I see it when I start the evening's shift. Her presence in the ER is so pronounced that I can always tell if I'm walking into a Sue-ER or non-Sue-ER. Her hostility and antagonism toward patients is legendary, especially to young mothers who bring their children into the ER for trivial reasons, like a snotty nose or fever of only one or two hours' duration. She's received reprimands time and again for bellowing at patients at triage when, in her opinion, they had no cause to be there. A stack of incident reports piled on the nurse manager's desk was rumored to be a foot high, not just from the patients whom she had treated or mistreated during their ER stay, but from fellow nurses and doctors she had pissed off. Not a few students and residents had been humiliated by Sue when they spoke to her in just the wrong way about some patient care issue — usually by telling her to do something that she had long since done, or by ordering labs, X rays, or other procedures that, once again in her estimation, they did not need.

The only reason she was still employed in the ER was that she was the best nurse to ever cross our doorway. She had been a pediatric nurse for ten or so years even before she arrived at our hospital, which was time immemorial, and there was nothing she did not know. She had a better eye for the subtle clues of illness than many attendings, and her long years of tending to people's needs had given her a sixth sense of distinguishing between what patients asked for and what they really needed. All the doctors there knew this, and so we all tolerated tirades and occasional abuse. She was hell on anyone she did not know or trust — she was pretty tough on those she did like — but once she knew you, and you knew *her,* things went pretty smoothly.

It was Friday, and the sense of portent was very, very strong. A polite Korean man walked by with a plastic cup from a fast-food chain. His age was indeterminate, somewhere between thirty and sixty. He was dressed carefully in shabby, threadbare clothes. Around his neck was a pair of headphones connected to a Walkman. I could hear the sound of Nirvana singing "hello . . . hello . . .

hello . . . hello." I watched him amusedly as he walked by, and I knew he was going to approach me the moment he saw me looking at him and making eye contact.

"Ah yu doctah?" he asked.

"Yes, do you need to be seen?" I said.

"Yu doctahs ah so brillian," he said. He grinned at me, as if he had just shared a great secret. Okay, I thought to myself, this guy is a nut. "I think yu doctah help me," he said.

I directed him to triage, and felt a little sorry for him. He was frail, and from the calm, direct way he looked at me, I assumed he must be pretty gentle, as well. Sue was at triage and she was not in a good mood, even for her. She was going to eat him alive. I glanced at the board behind my shoulder to see if there was a free room where I could just sit and talk with him for a minute and possibly get rid of him that way. No luck. All the rooms were full. So off he went to triage with his headphones trailing the voice of Kurt Cobain bellowing "I feel stupid and contagious . . ."

Forty-five minutes or so later I picked up a chart of a Mr. Kim who was forty-eight years old and had abdominal pain. It was my Korean guy. He smiled as if he could not believe his luck to be in my august presence again. "Oh, Doctah!" He warmly shook my hand and beamed again at me. "Yu brillian doctah. I know," and he nodded seriously.

"Thank you," I said. "I thought that only my mom had that kind of faith in me. What exactly is wrong with you today?"

He was not at all easy to understand, and it took a few minutes to figure out what the problem was. He held the cup up to me. He wanted it tested for poison.

"You want *what?*" I said.

He leaned closer to me, and it was clear he was trusting me with a great confidence. This was as comic a situation as I had seen for a long time, but his creepy, intense seriousness made me feel uncomfortable. "I don' have no sec drive," he said, his voice just above a whisper. "I drink this drink, and my sec drive is gone." He held the cup again for me to take.

I took a step backward. "Yu take this and yu brillian doctah can to know what poison I got," he insisted.

"How do you know it's poison?" I asked inanely.

Once again he leaned close to me. "My peen get small," he said, and looked at his pants for emphasis. "Yu give me pill, it give me back my sec drive," he said, nodding, as if there was not a trace of doubt that I knew which pill to give him to restore his penis and sex drive.

I went to triage to see if Sue had been able to figure out anything more about this fruitcake. I hoped that by a stroke of luck she knew Mr. Kim like she knew some of our other regulars, and would tell me what this particular delusion was all about. She was talking quietly to the social worker, who was nodding and making notes. There were two patients sitting just outside triage, a teenage boy and girl, or perhaps only one was the patient. The girl carried a shoebox.

"Hey, Sue, what's the deal with Mr. Kim?" I asked. Sue continued telling the social worker her story. "Hey, Sue?" I said again.

"Leave me alone right now, Joe, okay?" she barked.

This was Sue, after all; it was in her repertory. I hung around for a couple of minutes to listen. I didn't want to wait too long because Mr. Kim was clearly delusional and therefore potentially violent. That's just the way it is with nuts. But, as I listened, I realized the story Sue was telling the social worker clearly took precedence.

The girl was fifteen years old and had been brought in by her boyfriend because he was worried about her. She was having cramps for the past two or three days and wasn't eating. When they first came in, Sue said, she sent the boyfriend to the waiting room and had to argue with him to get him to leave. The girl, a pale, pretty, blond thing, wouldn't talk to her, and stared at the floor at her feet, clutching the box close to her.

Sue had asked her if this had anything to do with what was in the box. The girl shook her head and started to cry again. "I can't help you if you don't talk to me," Sue had told her, and just then the boyfriend tapped on the partition.

Sue pointed him back toward the waiting room, thinking that maybe he had beaten her up, or that perhaps the guy was her brother, not the boyfriend as she had assumed, and that she wouldn't talk with him around. He had mentioned cramps, so Sue suspected she might be having a miscarriage. She tried again for a few minutes, and again the girl remained tearful and mute, un-communicative. The guy was hovering outside again, and Sue decided that since she wasn't getting anywhere with the girl she would talk to him to find out what was going on.

"Who are you?" she had asked, and he told her that he was the girl's boyfriend. She was right in guessing that the girl was preg-nant, he told her. There was a tear in his eye. He had only found out two weeks ago, and she wanted to get an abortion. They had heard it was easier to get an abortion in the next state, so they put their money together and took a bus across the river to go to the clinic last week. Only they found when they got there that they didn't have enough cash, so they had to turn around and go home.

I looked at the kid again. He, too, was pale, but just as young and vulnerable looking as the girl. A few scraggly hairs grew under his chin, which must have made him seem old to his friends but only emphasized, to me, his baby face.

They tracked down another rumor that said that at a different clinic in another farther town, about eighty miles away, they would be able to get it done for free. They still had their money for the bus tickets — and sure enough, they were able to get into the clinic for free. The doctor at the clinic who examined her told them that she was too far gone to have an abortion: She was at least five months pregnant and he wasn't going to do it.

I thought of Mr. Kim, waiting for me to give him his pill to restore his penis and his sex drive. I didn't want to miss the end of the story, though.

Sue did something, and it took me a minute to figure out what she had done. She wiped a tear from her eye. And then the social worker did something I would never have thought to do: She laid a hand on her arm to comfort Sue. "Go ahead, tell me the rest."

They returned home, Sue said, and talked to their friends again, who told them that back in the sixties girls used to stick a coat hanger inside themselves to get rid of unwanted babies. The boyfriend said that he was against it but the girl had insisted she wasn't having no baby. So she untwisted a coat hanger and stuck it inside herself, and turned it a couple of times, and then she delivered a dead baby a couple of hours later. She put it in a shoebox. The boyfriend hadn't been there when she did it. That had been two days ago. She had stopped talking or eating, and he saw that she was bleeding. She wouldn't let him take her out of her bedroom. She fell asleep, and that's when he loaded her into his car and drove her to the ER. She woke up on the way in, and still said nothing, but clutched at the box.

We all involuntarily looked over at the two of them. I couldn't see the box, and I could barely make out their faces. The social worker said she would contact the teen-welfare services and left.

I had forgotten all about Mr. Kim by that time. Sue, the social worker, and I had decided that we needed to put the girl into one of the rooms in the back, and try to get her to let us examine her — she might have lost a lot of blood, and would, undoubtedly, sooner or later develop a serious uterine infection. I hoped Sue and the social worker could come up with an approach that would get the girl to trust us and let us help her.

I still had no idea what to do with Mr. Kim, and I had, in truth, lost interest. As I pulled the curtain to the Korean's room, I entered with an apology. "I'm sorry I kept you waiting so long — "

JULIAN ORENSTEIN, M.D.

"Yu doctah ah so stupid," he said, and he was as angry as he had been respectful earlier. The noisy music of Nirvana was emerging from his headphones again: "With the lights out it's less dangerous. Here we are now, entertain us!" Before I had a chance to say anything he stood up and glared at me. "Yu can't to know about no poison. I know. Yu doctah stupid."

I was taken aback. "Hold on, Mr. Kim. What's the problem? I had to take care of someone else, and that's why it took so long. Have a seat."

He looked at me uncertainly, then he did sit down.

"Good. Tell me again about the poison."

"I don' have no sec drive," he said. He nodded toward the cup. "I drink this drink, and my sec drive is gone. My peen get small," he said. Reluctantly he gave me the cup.

I looked down into it. It was not just empty, it was dry. Clean. Like it had not ever been used at all. "When did you drink the poison?" I said.

He waved his hand in dismissal at me and made a face, disparaging my ignorance. "Lon' ago." He clucked his tongue and said once again, "Yu can't to know about no poison. I know. Yu doctah stupid." He took his cup back and he walked out.

The boy was sitting outside the room where they had put his girlfriend. I put my hand on his shoulder. "You doin' okay?" I asked him. He nodded his head. He seemed vacant, the kind of kid I would never have given a second thought about, but he had just shown his true colors in a very impressive way. "What's her name?" I asked.

"Stephanie."

"Is that how you call her?"

"I call her Steph."

Steph. I went in. She was sitting on the bed in the middle of the room. She had left the box on the counter, a foot or two away. I hadn't expected that. I introduced myself, and told her that the nurse and her boyfriend had already filled me in on a lot of what had happened. The overhead lights had been turned off, and the side lamp gave the room a soft, almost cozy lighting. She was dressed in a gown, and I marveled that Sue had convinced her to get that far.

She was staring downward, as she had been outside triage. When I spoke she flicked her eyes up in my direction, and then looked down. She nodded her head in acknowledgment of what I had said.

"Steph, I need to look you over and make sure you're all right."

Once again she nodded in a barely perceptible way.

"I would also like to look at your baby."

Then, for the first time she looked straight at me. She could not decide whether to trust me or not. "No, you can't do that," she said, and looked at the box. This was the first time she had spoken to anyone. A minor victory.

"Here," I said, "you can hold it." Her eyes darted anxiously as I picked up the shoebox and handed it to her.

It felt empty.

I was so startled by the lack of weight, that I shook it to make sure, and reached to open the lid, only she got to it first, and pulled it tight against her belly.

"Is your baby in there?" I asked. But the opportunity had been lost. She was not going to talk to me again. She gathered her gown around herself and slid past me, and in a swift motion, picked up her pile of clothes and backed away into a corner of the room.

"You could be developing a serious infection. You may have lost a lot of blood," I said. I was pleading with her. It did no good. She just shook her head. "You have to let us help you."

I stood there for another minute. Somehow Sue and the social worker had gotten her in there; maybe they could undo some of the damage I had done. I left to find them, and, of course, when we got back she was gone, and so was her boyfriend.

JULIAN ORENSTEIN, M.D.

I told Sue and the social worker about how the box had felt empty, and they didn't believe me. "Why would she have brought in an empty box?" Sue asked me.

"Why did Mr. Kim bring in an empty cup? Who knows why people do half of the things they do?" I replied.

It was late, and it was the end of our shifts. We were on the ambulance dock, and Sue was smoking. I watched the curls of smoke rising. "What did you come to find me for in the first place?" she asked.

"Never mind," I said. "Never mind."

BODY PACKER

BY *Barry Pollack, M.D.*

I joined two men, each over six foot, strong and burly, as they accompanied the teenager into the elevator. It was an old elevator, whose cables creaked and strained to lift its passengers, at one agonizingly slow speed to the top floor. The makers of this building were practical, not superstitious. And so the top floor was the thirteenth. The building was Los Angeles County Hospital — a major medical center and teaching hospital.

On the thirteenth floor, the elevator doors opened into a waiting room. The walls were white but had a sickly greenish hue from overhead fluorescents in wire-caged fixtures. There were several dial-less phones hanging on the wall, which visitors used to speak to patients separated from them by a thick glass window. A steel-barred, electrically locked sliding door led into the ward. The patients inside were not in medical isolation. They were prisoners. The thirteenth floor was the county jail's emergency ward.

The tall, strong men were police officers. The pimply teen was my patient and their prisoner. Exiting the elevator, the two cops nonchalantly nodded to one of their compatriots who guarded the entrance to the jail ward. And with no more security than that nod, the barred doors opened.

My patient was eighteen, with a peach-fuzzed and blemished face, newly arrived from Colombia. He had been seen at a private hospital earlier in the day, complaining of severe abdominal pain. As part of his evaluation, X rays were taken that showed twenty small, round objects in his bowel. Each was the size of a walnut. Panicked that he was going to die, the boy admitted to smuggling drugs by swallowing small balloons filled with cocaine: a "body packer." He planned to retrieve them when they passed in his stool. The police arrested him. What they wanted from me was not a diagnosis. They had the diagnosis. What they wanted was evidence.

The medical concern was what to do about the multiple foreign bodies that my young patient had swallowed. Coins, marbles, and dentures are often swallowed and pass through the bowel uneventfully. It was expected that these "balloons" too would pass. I did, however, have to explain one particular risk to my patient.

"If just one of those balloons bursts, spilling cocaine into your gut, . . . you will die."

My patient eyed me bewilderedly.

"*Comprende?*" I asked.

He understood all right. But this was never part of his plan. Smuggling drugs was supposed to be a route to riches, not death. Certainly not death.

My young drug smuggler pleaded. It was the first time he'd done this, he said. He didn't want to die. Wasn't there something I could do? The cops were amused. Every prisoner in jail has the same story. They either didn't do it (an MMOB: "minding my own business"), or it was the first time.

"*No es culpa mía,*" the boy said over and over. It's not my fault. That was probably the greatest fault of all the thieves, murderers, drug dealers, and other sordid types we treated on the jail ward. No one could admit blame. Someone else or some unfortunate life event was always at fault for their crime. But not them.

Body Packer

213

Although you couldn't help but become jaded somewhat by the despicable characters you found as patients on jail ward, the cops had one job, I had another. They were jailers, I was a doctor. Their job was to keep order. Mine was to offer remedy and compassion.

I consulted the surgeons. "He's got a benign belly right now," the surgical resident told me. "Just opening him up could pose significant risk." So the surgeons, unwilling to operate, were unhelpful.

I consulted Internal Medicine. "No," the internist said, "you don't want to give laxatives or cathartics to encourage quick passage of the balloons. Vigorous peristalsis might cause the balloons to burst." They passed on the case too.

And I consulted Gastroenterology. "No," the GI resident confirmed what I already suspected. "Trying to grab hold of those balloons with an endoscope would likely perforate the rubber. And that'd be that."

And so this patient was mine, and mine alone. The only solution was to wait, hope for the best, and prepare for the worst.

The police, concerned that my body packer might pass his contraband and flush the evidence away, would not allow him to be in one of the regular locked rooms on the ward. His ankles were cuffed to a gurney and he was parked in the middle of the hall — better to keep an eye on him. An emergency crash cart was at his bedside, just in case. He had an intravenous line in each arm, electrodes on his chest, and a cardiac monitor at his feet. He had no books, no magazines, no music, and no friendly company. His gaze could fall only upon the ominously quiet tracing of his heartbeat on the cardiac monitor, or the bemused, uncompassionate, and equally ominous stare of nearby cops.

I always felt safe on the jail ward, certainly safer than in the emergency room. The ER had a track record for violence perpetrated against doctors and staff. There, an irate patient frustrated by too long a wait could decide to shoot up the place; or some gangbanger might walk in flailing a knife, seeking to complete his vengeance upon one of our patients; or some violent wacko, doped out on alcohol or drugs, could hop off a gurney and go on a rampage. We didn't have metal detectors because hospital administrators were concerned about the *image* it would send to the community. *Image!*

So unlike the ER, the jail ward was a safe haven. Though a history of aberrant behavior was the norm for patients here, no foul-mouthed, belligerent, or uncooperative attitudes were tolerated on the thirteenth floor. I may have heard "Screw you, Doc" from a patient once, . . . but rarely twice. Any patients who mouthed off or just looked at me wrong found themselves succumbing to half a dozen officers, who "did their duty" in an instant. Although we were in a hospital, our patients were all reminded that it was jail, too, with locked rooms, armed cops, and quick retribution.

L.A. County is the last resort for medical care of those who well know it is their last resort. And for those in training, it provides a cornucopia of maladies to learn from. Sure there were plenty of other wards where a medical resident could serve; but none was a better teaching ground for medicine, nor a better mirror on life than the thirteenth floor. And, perhaps more than any other place in our society, the jail ward was one place where justice triumphed. Our legal system often seems to fail in providing the guilty with their just deserts. Attorneys have turned the concepts of law and justice into antitheses. They delay, wrangle, and bargain, more often obscuring justice rather than serving it. But on the jail ward, one frequently finds that biblical justice has prevailed.

On the thirteenth floor you could find the drive-by shooter street gangster who had a permanent colostomy after a gunshot wound to his belly, the bank robber paralyzed after crashing his getaway car, the liquor store thief whose right hand was shot off by his partner who missed while blasting away with a shotgun at the store owner, and of course, a drug smuggler threatened with death by an overdose of his own contraband.

I still remember how my body packer looked each time his stomach spasms recurred. The cardiac monitor would blare a shrill warning as the slow, steady rhythm of his heart gave way to a racing beat brought on by pain. His face contorted and he wept, not so much from pain as from fear, as he waited to either pass the evidence that would put him in jail or feel his heart give out.

Plato said, "It is right that a wicked man be punished as a sick man be cured; for all punishment is a kind of medicine." And so we served both medicine and justice on the jail ward.

Several months after my experience on the thirteenth floor, I had another young patient. Not unlike my Colombian body packer, he was also in his teens. And though perhaps better bred and richer born, he suffered from that same youthful and baleful attitude that he could have all the world had to give by just wanting it, but without earning it.

I met him in a private hospital. One whose patients were well insured, more affluent, and one far from any thirteenth floor. He wore expensive boots and those trendy jeans with the knees torn out that make looking poor snobbish. His legs were rubbery, his face was pasty and fearful as two friends carried him into the emergency room and laid him on a gurney. They disappeared a moment later before any questions could be asked. So much for friends.

"What's the matter?" I asked. There was no evidence of trauma, no blood.

"My heart's beatin' out of my chest," he answered. "Am I gonna die, Doc?"

He dripped sweat, his pupils were dilated the size of dimes, and his heart raced as if he'd just run a marathon. He admitted to doing "speedballs," a combination of cocaine and heroin. Looking for a euphoric high, he instead discovered the other effects of cocaine — anxiety, depression, confusion, dizziness, headaches, and fear.

We started an IV and put him on a cardiac monitor. Though his vital signs were stable, cardiovascular collapse and dangerous heart rhythms are common with cocaine abuse. We gave him IV medication to slow his heart rate and a Valium to calm his anxiety.

As he felt better and his fear and discomfort dissipated, I felt too that his fear of using cocaine again would be short-lived.

"I've done crack, ice, speed, lots of other stuff, and this kinda thing never happened to me before," he explained. He was not apologetic nor regretful. He was matter-of-fact. His brush with death was over. It was as if he had merely slipped on some path of ice in his life's path — unfortunate, but nothing to keep him from going on.

There's a whole vocabulary for drugs on the street. There's crack, rock, snow, blow, toot, ice, bernice, lady, champagne, and baseball. But no matter what you call it, it's poison. And it's not just the young experimenting with drugs. It's the affluent and well-educated crowd as well. People that wouldn't stoop to eat a morsel of food that had fallen on the floor don't think twice about snorting, smoking, or injecting drugs concocted by nefarious dealers in vermin-infested garages and mixed with heroin, amphetamines, talc, corn starch, anything handy. And do they think where it comes from?

"Do you know where coke comes from?" I asked my patient. He shrugged his shoulders, disinterested.

"It comes out of the asses of young men like you. And then you sniff it up your nose. It comes from young men like you who find themselves dying in a bathroom looking for riches in a toilet bowl."

I was angry. I knew he didn't care. But I told him anyway about my patient on the thirteenth floor. I tell all my "dopers" the story. Just maybe somebody will listen.

MENINGOCOCCUS

BY *Susan Mates, M.D.*

Listen. She is a lily among thorns, curls luster like black grapes, lips a scarlet thread. She lies, her plump baby arms held down, on the white table and screams. We see her ripe cheeks, the flowers of the earth, the singing of birds. Her parents stand off by the open doors of the ambulance bay and watch.

Her feet are beautiful and chubby, skin the palest pink, veiled in tiny purple dots. She was fine an hour ago. Her thighs are firm, creased with bursting fullness. The dots became blotches. We stare, the nurses, the resident, and I, and puncture the ivory of her arms with needles. I am the intern and innocent. I have not yet seen a child die.

We barely speak, we work so fast. She stops crying, now just whimpering, soon she doesn't resist at all. The purple spreads, her belly, her navel, she is pooling, coalescing, darkening. Her eyes consider us. They are blue, the eyes of doves by the rivers of water, washed with tears and milk. Her mother should be taken away. She stands, her lips parted, staring, a pillar of salt. Her father covers his face. There is no one to go to them. We are consumed by the child. We force a plastic tube through her sweet mouth, her teeth are a flock of sheep. We tilt her silken head back, we pump her mottled chest. Our love, our little sister.

We push, we breathe, we stab, we take blood and give penicillin, and still we do not stop or think. One of us, a nurse, holds the tiny intravenous in place with one hand while the other hand idly strokes the girl's hair. She does this without thinking. The electrocardiogram runs. The baby's eyes have rolled up into her long lashes. Where has she gone? To the garden, the bed of spices, the gathered lilies. We adults, doctors, have not watched. Foxes, that is our guilt from this moment on, the little foxes that spoil the vines.

The line is flat now, it has been for some time. We cannot believe, we refuse to stop. We push, and breathe, and now, we weep. She has set a seal on our heart, she has branded us, even though the time can be counted in seconds, minutes. We pull the curtain. We do not speak. The oldest of us is only twenty-seven and when she tells the parents what they already know, her tongue will turn to stone. When we have children of our own, we will trust nothing, our vigilance relentless.

Run, lovely little one, and be like a young deer on the mountain. We wrap your tiny body in coarse white sheets. Love is as strong as death and as cruel as the grave. Your parents will never recover.

Meningococcus

DAY ONE

BY *Michael Palmer, M.D.*

nternship. They call it first-year residency most places now, perhaps serving the dual purpose of assuaging some of the fear in the patients . . . and in the fledgling docs. But back in the late sixties it was internship. I did mine on the Harvard Medical Service at the Boston City Hospital. And my first rotation was in the ER.

It was the last year before Lyndon Johnson's Great Society program created Medicare and Medicaid, making private patients out of many of the poor and disenfranchised who previously had no place to go but City. Suddenly, Mass General, New England Medical Center, the Peter Bent Brigham, and all the rest of the upper-crust Boston hospitals would be competing for patients they used to put in vacuum tubes to shoot across town to that gritty old place on Harrison Avenue. Over time, the Boston City ER census would drop by almost two-thirds, although it remained and still remains a "zoo" much of the time. Inpatient wards would close. At some point, the full-time police station located in the ER would shut down as well.

But when I put my name tag on my freshly laundered, hyper-starched, white clinic coat and walked through the doors of the ER for my first shift, politics and impending social change were light-years from my mind. Every fact I had ever learned seemed to be in competition to dominate my thoughts. And I was scared stiffer than that coat.

I went to Case Western Reserve University School of Medicine in Cleveland, which is a wonderful place to go to med school. But Case had always been a very cerebral sort of school that stressed techniques of interviewing over performing procedures such as spinal taps, and perfecting diagnostic deduction and case synthesis over seeing hundreds of different kinds of patients. The truth is, internship is a great equalizer. And within a week or two, everyone had learned as much as everyone else about surviving and growing as a doc at Boston City.

For me, my first day in the ER was about all it took to reach that point.

I had spent the three weeks between my med school graduation and that first day in a smoldering state of panic. Textbooks and notes on ER medicine covered every table and most of the floor space in our new apartment. I was twenty-five years old, and the bulk of my life experience to that point had consisted of school and summer camp. Because I did my surgical clerkship at a VA hospital, I had never worked in an ER. And by the luck of the draw, none of the patients I was assigned in any of my med school clerkships had died. I actually choose Boston City because I wanted a rough-and-tumble internship to complement the more theoretical training at Case.

Now, on that warm July morning, as I crossed the deserted ambulance bay and entered the ER, it was time to stand by that decision.

Just stay cool . . . just stay cool . . .

The words, a continuous mantra in my brain during those three weeks of preparation, droned on like white noise as I picked up a chart from the rack and went in to see my first patient as a licensed physician.

Just stay cool. . . . No matter what happens, stay cool and think . . .

I was assigned to Dick Garibaldi, the resident in charge, to cover Rooms 1, 2, 3, and 4 on the male medical wing of the ER. The uses of the rooms changed depending on what the nurses needed, but basically, 1 and 2 were for "routine" cases. Room 4 was for major medical — cardiac arrests and the like — and 3 was for the alcoholics and other down-and-outers, many of whom considered the ER staff family.

My first patient was a young man with a sore throat. During my excessive workup on him, I am certain Garibaldi treated a dozen or more patients on the other wing. At last, the cultures and the tests for mono and hypothyroidism and God only knows what else were off to the lab. I wrote a prescription for penicillin and sent the man on his way with a detailed follow-up plan.

One sick person, one perfect work-up, one probable cure, I said to myself. What in the hell had I been so worried about all these weeks, anyway?

"Um, Dr. Palmer," the nurse said quietly, patiently, "you may want to go a little bit faster. There are two patients in Room Two, six in Room Three."

By nine o'clock, the beginning of hour two of my first day, I discovered I had another gear and saw three times as many patients as I had in hour one. By the end of that second hour, I was so far behind that Garibaldi began seeing patients on his side and mine to help me catch up.

By ten, I had discovered a higher gear still. I found it by accepting that in the ER at least, all of those Case Western Reserve interview techniques I had practiced so diligently were useless . . . or worse. One of my patients that hour was an elderly woman, dropped off on the ER by somebody who then left without speaking to any of us. The history, written on her chart by our intake worker, read, "found in a linen closet."

A few minutes later, another woman, named Margaret, an angelic-faced octogenarian, arrived by ambulance in a fairly deep coma. She had a temperature of 105 and evidence of septic shock. Her five sons trooped in behind the litter. They all lived at home.

"Hey, guys, can you tell me what's going on here?"

"You know, Doc, it was the funniest thing. We were just sitting there in the living room having tea with mother when the ambulance came and took her away."

A concerned neighbor, apparently also invited for tea, had called. Eventually, Margaret recovered from her aspiration pneumonia and returned home to her sons, who, hopefully, observed her a bit more carefully before feeding her.

Eleven o'clock. Another hour, another gear. Garibaldi had returned to working only his side. The nurses and I were beginning to function with a certain rhythm and harmony. My pulse was beginning to slow to a sublethal level. Then it happened. A police officer burst through the ER doors, pushing a litter ahead of him. On the litter was a man — the sickest human being I had ever seen. The officer, clearly familiar with the ER, charged straight into Room 4. One of the nurses and I followed. The nurse and cop began cutting his clothes off. I stood several feet away, silently screaming the litany which had been muted throughout most of the frantic morning.

Just stay cool. . . . Keep your cool and think about what you learned in physical diagnosis. . . . Do you auscultate, then palpate, then percuss? Or do you palpate, then —

"Excuse me, Dr. Palmer," the nurse called over her shoulder, "but this man's not breathing."

Aha! That's why the guy looked so terrible. He wasn't breathing. The report galvanized me into action.

"Blow your whistle," I ordered.

The ER was so vast that each of the nurses had a whistle hanging from her stethoscope to call for help. This particular nurse had seen her share of July firsts, hesitated just a beat, then shrugged and blew. Footsteps . . . excited voices . . . the clattering of rolling wheels. . . . My first Code 99. The ultimate ER experience. Nurses, orderlies, and technicians spilled into Room 4. I started toward the patient but kept glancing toward the door for Garibaldi. He arrived in just a few seconds, but by the time he charged in, the staff was milling about like restless cattle, waiting for some sort of order from someone. They stepped aside as he headed for the litter. I moved in behind him to assist . . . and to learn.

At the bedside, Garibaldi stopped short. Then he raised the man's arm off the mattress and let it go. It stayed in that position. Right there. Rigor mortis. The guy had been dead for at least a day, maybe two. That's why he looked so terrible. Rigidity . . . dependent lividity . . . back half deep purple, front half yellow green . . . all were definitely grim prognostic signs.

"Palmer, did you touch him? Did you *touch* him?" Garibaldi's voice was an octave or two higher than usual.

To my right, two nurses, laughing too hard to stand, slid to the floor, tears welling.

"You gotta *touch* him, Palmer," Garibaldi went on, making no attempt to quiet the nurses in the corner. "You absolutely have to touch him. If he's room temperature, you gotta suspect this isn't gonna work. Never depend on the police, or anyone else for that matter, to tell you what's going on."

Garibaldi was one of the legends around the hospital. Dedicated, tireless, creative, unflappable, and smart as hell. Now, I knew, I was about to become something of a legend myself. By the time my shift was over, there wouldn't be a dietary or maintenance worker who hadn't heard about the Code 99 the new intern called on an absolute stiff.

"Dr. Palmer," the nurse said as the room emptied out. "We're about twenty patients behind." Head down, looking for a giant hole, I started off. She put her arm around my shoulder. "Hey, don't worry, you'll do fine."

"Yeah . . . sure. Thanks."

I glanced up at one of the ubiquitous wall clocks. It was noon.

Over the next three hours, perhaps by an act of Providence, there was something of a lull. With Garibaldi's help, I began to get caught up. There was a Code 99 on his wing, the real deal this time. The patient made it, and I actually contributed. The next morning I would run a code myself, and later that day, I would do one with two nurses. No whistles.

But day one wasn't over for me just yet. And what was, perhaps, the biggest single lesson of my life in medicine was awaiting me in Room 3.

The chart said his name was Robert. I can't remember his last name. Age fifty-one. Chief complaint, headaches. A grizzled down-and-outer with oil-stained clothes, and a hollowness between the bones of his hands that was mirrored in his eyes. He had been sitting there patiently, in no particular distress, as one by one I dealt with each of the other men in Room 3. Finally, there were just the two of us. It was only then, as I took his chart from the rack and turned to him, that I realized he stank. It was an odor unlike any I had ever encountered — a heavy, fetid, sad stench that would keep all but the most intrepid caregivers at arm's length.

But this was still day one for me. It was too late in the afternoon to send Robert over to the walk-in clinic. And I was too new to know which medical shortcuts were safe to take. If one of our two orderlies wasn't too engrossed in the racing form, perhaps he would agree to help Robert get into a johnny for an examination. It seemed possible that with his clothes sealed in a plastic bag, it might be easier to get close.

Tiso, the orderly, reluctantly agreed to help me out.

I wrote a few charts and tried to believe that the giggles coming from the nurses' station next door had nothing to do with a certain

Code 99. I reminded myself that with my first day on the ER winding down, the only one who had been seriously damaged by my performance was me.

Five minutes should be enough even for Tiso. I headed back to Room 3, glancing down the other wing as I passed. Garibaldi was examining a male patient on a stretcher in the hall. All of his rooms were in action. I wondered if a year ago some resident had been forced to carry him. Doubtful.

I took two or three steps into Room 3 and froze. Robert, dressed only in a robin's-egg blue johnny, his grease-stained Red Sox cap, and paper booties, looked at me impassively. If he felt as ridiculous as he looked, he hid it well. The devastating smell was, to all intents, unchanged. And in that moment, I knew why. On his left lower leg, extending from just below his knee to just above his ankle, was a deep raw ulcer. And covering most of the ulcer was a wriggling white sheet of maggots.

Nothing in my suburban upbringing, or my comparative anatomy, or my YMCA summer camp, or organic chemistry had prepared me for that moment. I handled the jet of bile and wave of nausea reasonably well, but it was as if Medusa was sitting there in a johnny. I could not look directly at the man or his leg.

"Um . . . ah . . . sir," I managed between glances at the ceiling, floor, door, and walls. "I . . . I don't know if you know it or not, but there's a huge ulcer on the front of your leg and . . . it'scrawlingtoptobottomwithmaggots!"

Robert looked down at his leg, then up at the earnest boy in the starched white coat. From somewhere within the dark hollows, his eyes sparked. But otherwise he remained unfazed. Finally, he sighed. His expression was one of a Nobel physicist about to try and explain relativity to a junior high science class.

"Son," he said, glancing down once more at his leg, then at me, "everyone on my block has one of these. . . . But they don't all have these goddamn headaches!"

Robert spent that night as a patient on the Harvard Medical Service. I spent it passed out facedown on top of the bedspread. I heard that his leg responded well to treatment and that his headaches got better after repair of his bleeding stomach ulcer helped correct his severe anemia. All in all, he was in Boston City for about two weeks. I doubt he gave a second thought to the kid who admitted him. But twenty-seven years later that kid still remembers him well.

THE GARDENER

BY *Siegfried Kra, M.D.*

Bill was employed by a computer firm, but his real ambition was to become a gardener. He was a tall, pale, young man with eyes as black as coal. He had long delicate hands like a pianist, hands that looked like they had not been used for physical labor. With some trepidation I hired him to take care of the grounds.

At the end of the day as the sun set, he arrived in a Jeep Cherokee driven by a young woman. She was a tall, slender thing with long, brown hair, her eyes as dark as two amethyst jewels, with the features of a gently carved Grecian goddess. She carried a small book. Side by side, the two of them held hands, like they were posing for one of Picasso's blue period paintings.

"I'll wait until you finish," I heard her say in a soft, gentle voice. She handed him fruit and a small canteen. "It's very warm. Drink, or you'll sweat and feel weak."

He kissed her gently on the lips and proceeded to find his way to the toolshed. She sat in the Jeep, in the darkness, patiently waiting for him.

Bill liked to work until the late evening, unperturbed by the darkness.

"Why work at night, and so late?" I asked him.

"It's cooler. The ground is soft and moist at night; it makes digging and planting easier."

He wore torn dungarees, a red handkerchief around his forehead, and a polo shirt. He began to look more and more like a gardener each night.

He did a splendid job, this nocturnal gardener of mine. Once, when a dangerous thunderstorm arrived, soaking the dry earth from weeks of torrid heat, he continued digging, planting unperturbed that his body was drenched from the rain. His girlfriend sat languidly in the Jeep Cherokee in the darkness, waiting for him.

From my window, I saw him place the garden tools in the shed, raise his head to the sky, catching the rain in his open mouth, and then walk slowly over to the vehicle. The young woman wiped his face with a towel as if he had just stepped out of a shower. She placed her slender arms around his soaked body, her lips on his cheek and they departed.

What a strange couple. They hardly spoke but her eyes were always fastened on him.

He planted flowers that I had never seen. My once pitiful, listless garden soon gleamed with a kaleidoscope of rich colors. The young gardener looked on with pride like an artist who created beauty on a canvas.

Each week he presented me with a modest bill, and made more suggestions about how to further beautify the grounds around my house.

"You have a charming young friend," I said to him. "She is welcome to rest inside. She need not sit out there alone in the dark."

"No, she likes to sit in the Jeep to listen to the wind and the trees."

Each day I waited for the gardener, hoping to catch a glimpse of his mysterious young woman. Every night she drove the Jeep to the far side of the driveway. Then she gave him a red silk scarf and tied it around his head, adjusting it carefully so it did not cover his eyes.

"You must come during the day sometimes, to see the colors of the garden," I told the young woman. "Your boyfriend did such a splendid job."

"I don't have to see the flowers. I can feel and smell the flowers, especially at night when the fragrance is so much keener. Though, perhaps, one day I will."

"Are you a student?" I asked.

I knew she did not want to speak to me, but I persisted. "You look like an art student or an English major."

"Neither. I work as a receptionist at the place where my boyfriend works," she replied. "I used to go to school," she said proudly, unashamed that now she was a receptionist in the computer company just to be near her lover.

One night the cold and warm air met, covering my house with a thick fog. A full moon was reflecting eerie shadows on the garden. It was late, and I surrendered to the night. I figured the lovers wouldn't come that night. Then the lights of the Jeep streamed through the fog. I was in bed, and watched the beautiful scene unfold through the open window.

She undressed in the darkness, in the moonlight, and danced her naked feet around the flowers, raising her long, slender arms to the moon. I caught a glimpse of her radiant body in the bright, shimmering blue light. She became a goddess of the night, and her lover was now at her side. He placed flowers in her hair that he picked from the garden. They never touched, as if she was too sacred to be touched by anything human. A cloud circled the moon, the fog returned. When the dance was over, she tiptoed back to the Jeep. He followed. The Jeep moved out of the driveway leaving a magic behind that had never been there before.

The scene unnerved me for days. Perhaps it was all a dream, an illusion. Perhaps the garden now did have magical power that the strange, beautiful woman brought into my life. The garden looked more beautiful than before.

The gardener suddenly stopped coming. Days passed and not one word from him. At first I became annoyed, then anger gave way to melancholy. At least he should have had the decency to call if he no longer wanted to work. He did not even bother to collect his salary. Each night I waited, skipping any engagements. Just to sit by the window looking, waiting. Sleepless nights followed one another. The image of the young woman dancing naked in the garden never left me.

Finally, I relinquished my pride, as a disappointed lover, and I made the call. He was at home and he answered the phone in his usual ethereal voice.

"I will be there tomorrow, Doctor, I promise," he said. "I was tied up a little."

No apologies, no explanations. It was not important for him to give any explanation to an old man. I expected him to arrive in the early evening, but instead he arrived alone in the middle of the morning the following day.

"Where is your girlfriend?" I asked with consternation in my voice. I wanted to tell him how I watched their moonlight dance, and how the garden became special, magical, by her touch, her breath on the flowers. He must have sensed my disappointment.

"We broke up" was all he said.

His face was listless and he no longer seemed interested in his work.

He came during the day, in the torrid sun. His movements slowed and the garden lost its magical beauty. He neglected to weed, water, and before long the garden looked unattractive, neglected. I dared not say anything to him. His eyes were red and swollen as if he no longer slept. He was moving as if he was walking in a dream, going through the motions of being alive.

"What happened?" I asked him.

The Gardener

"It just happened. One day she said she no longer wanted me."

She had done her job well, this enchanted sorceress from another world, and then disappeared.

"You are so young and there are hundreds of women out there for you to meet," I said with no conviction in my voice. I understood and shared his pain because I, too, once felt his loss.

Several weeks later, I asked him to trim the bushes around the house. He refused the electric cutter and used an old pair of garden scissors. He worked at a feverish pace, sweating profusely, cutting and snipping as if he was carving out the pain he felt in his heart. Always in silence, rounding out all the bushes in perfect symmetry as a compulsive draftsman, completely oblivious to the throngs of hornets circling his head. He suddenly straightened his bent body, flinching with pain from dozens of bites. He dropped the scissors, desperately slapping hornets from his face and neck.

"Doctor," he called in a soft, hollow voice. "Can I see you for a minute?"

I was in my study, annoyed to be disturbed. Both of us lost interest in the garden, the grounds. Casually, nonchalantly, bored, I arrived at the porch door.

"Some hornets bit me and I'm allergic to them."

He looked frightened, his face was the color of mud. I suddenly awoke from my lethargy. I rushed to the medicine cabinet and found only Benadryl, which he swallowed swiftly.

"How do you feel?"

"Not so good. My lips are swelling, and my mouth feels like it is filled with cotton."

Right before my eyes, his arms and face grew flush and swollen, like a red balloon. He swayed like a drunken sailor as I guided him to my car.

"We have to hurry. There isn't much time."

I drove through traffic lights, beeping the horn, swinging my stethoscope out of the window, so they'd make way for me as I sped desperately to the emergency room. In the mirror I could see his ashen face. "How are you? Keep talking," I said to him, as if speaking would keep him alive.

"I can't breathe, I feel something heavy on my chest, everything is dark now, like somebody put a mask over my face." He fell back, I slammed on the brakes, jumped out of the car, breathed into his mouth, and pounded on his chest. The gardener stirred. There was no one there to help. Only curious gapers in passing cars. He suffered anaphylactic shock, a dreadful allergic reaction to hornet bites. One shot of adrenaline and he could be saved.

What stupidity on my part not to have at least adrenaline in my doctor's bag that lay covered with dust in the trunk of my car. That brown alligator bag given to me the day I started practice was once part of my professional dress. Once stuffed with medicines to save lives, now it lay covered with years of disuse, the drugs browned with decay, useless. My, how the practice of my art had changed. I used to carry it on daily house calls, a badge of trust that commanded respect even in the worst of neighborhoods: "There goes the doc, let him be."

If I had called an ambulance it might have taken ten, even fifteen minutes before they found the house. He might have died by his magical garden that he planted so lovingly. In minutes we were in the emergency room and I screamed into the hall, a scream of despair.

"I have a dying boy in my car, he had a swarm of hornets bite him." They carried him to the special room for patients with cardiac arrest. His face was ashen, his eyes opened. My job was done. Now the young physicians, certainly not as old as the gardener, were racing to save him. They must have seen themselves lying on the ground. How swiftly they moved, what expert reflexes, not one motion wasted as I stood there feeling old, helpless. This is a job for the young. I was a poor surrogate for the ambulance.

I called his mother, who at first did not understand. "Better come to the emergency room at once. Things are not going well."

"I don't drive," she said. "I'll have to call his friend to take me there."

They arrived like two sisters through the swinging door. His mother was erect and proud looking. A copy of her son, the same eyes, the same poetical face, even the same black shade of hair. The young woman with her, the goddess of the garden, was formally dressed. At first I wasn't sure she was the woman I saw dancing so freely in the moonlight. She carried a book with her, as if she was going to have a long wait ahead. She sat in the waiting room, her face expressionless, without a tinge of sadness.

She came here as the driver and nothing more. "He knew he was allergic to bees," she finally spoke. "He always carried his insect kit with him, right in his jeans pocket — look for yourself, it's still there . . ."

BAND MASTER

BY *Richard Haight, M.D.*

Doctor, University Hospital just called. The helicopter is leaving and will be here in half an hour. Do you want me to cancel some patients?"

"No thanks, Ruby. We're almost caught up, but call some of these people and warn them that we'll be running a little late due to the emergency." Dr. Roberts pointed to the growing appointment list as he spoke. An already hectic morning was becoming worse. As usual he had gotten up at six A.M. to round at the hospital. He was especially anxious to see how Johnny Thomas had spent the night. Roberts had pinned his fractured hip earlier that week, but the elderly farmer wasn't recovering well. The nurse had called during the night to express her concern that Johnny was having a stroke, but this morning's exam had confirmed Roberts's suspicion that Johnny was merely overmedicated. He discontinued all of his sedatives and pain medications. By evening Johnny would be more alert, although definitely more uncomfortable.

The real problem of the day had arrived in Emergency just before office hours. Jim Treadwell, the high school band director, was having a massive heart attack. It hadn't come as a total surprise to either Roberts or to Treadwell, whose brother and father had both succumbed to MI's in their forties. Jim's cholesterol level indicated that he would not be spared either. Despite this history, he had denied the chest pain after the school banquet last night, believing it to be heartburn. Like many others who deny the early warning signs of a heart attack, he had taken antacids and massaged his left arm throughout the night. His wife, June, called the ambulance when he collapsed at the breakfast table.

Fortunately he didn't live far from the hospital, and June, fearful of this inevitable event, had taken a Red Cross CPR class at the local library. He was still in ventricular fibrillation, however, when he hit the emergency room, his skin badly mottled from lack of oxygen. Roberts had acted quickly by passing an intubation tube down past the vocal cords and pumping oxygen into his lungs with an ambu bag. At the same time he snapped orders to the scurrying personnel to prepare for cardioversion and start an IV.

While a nurse took over the bagging, Roberts picked up the paddles and stood like a cymbal player awaiting his cue. Warning everyone to stand clear, he triggered the high voltage into Treadwell's chest. Treadwell's body spasmed briefly, then stopped. The monitor showed a flat line — no heartbeat. Anticipating his next command the nurse handed Roberts a long-needled syringe full of adrenaline. Roberts quickly palpated along the ribs with two fingers and plunged the needle through the chest wall into the heart. Dark blood started to fill the syringe, and at that same instant he injected the stimulant. "Come on," he pleaded while snapshots of the band master, a saxophone, and fellow students quaking in his wrath flashed through his mind. Moments later, as if on cue, the heart monitor began its characteristic beep and the nurse was able to register a blood pressure.

Dr. Roberts looked up and smiled wanly. As in the past, he dared not fail the man on the table. He ordered dopamine and TPA from the pharmacy. Tissue plasminogen activator was the new wonder drug that, if used within hours of chest pain onset, could dissolve the clot causing the heart attack. Roberts couldn't admit it was probably too late for the clot buster to work. The arrhythmia itself had already caused severe damage to Treadwell's heart, and very possibly his brain.

He stepped back from Jim Treadwell and for the first time noticed the pain and anguish in the faces around him. Everyone knew Jim, and most had been his student at one time or another. Like Roberts, they too had survived the fury of this man with the keen ear who knew every note each band member should play and demanded precision performances. He had taught in town for twenty-five years, creating bands that were legendary throughout the state. His program was rooted deep in the grade schools, and he was a magician when it came to turning an immature bunch of farm kids into a finely tuned concert band. The high school band was a great source of pride to the school, the community, and the surrounding countryside. If the farmers agreed on no other issue, they were unified at a Jim Treadwell concert.

Roberts hung the bag of TPA solution and began to calculate the flow rate for the dopamine drip. A nurse solemnly checked and rechecked the blood pressure. Roberts thought about his saxophone again. By the time he was in junior high he hated it, but his mother wouldn't let him quit. He would never forget his first solo experience squawking through *Solito Lindo,* his face burning with embarrassment. The other parents sat and smiled politely as they tried not to wince, but his mother tapped the cadence with her foot and beamed broadly.

It was to his astonishment that after playing for the great man himself he was the last eighth-grade saxophone chosen for the high school band. He was doubly surprised to learn that he would no longer be playing the alto but rather the baritone saxophone. His eyes widened at the sight of Mr. Treadwell holding an instrument as big as Roberts himself.

"It won't be as hard to play as it looks," assured Mr. Treadwell, and he was right. Despite its size, a small breath of air created a deep, rich bass sound and for Roberts it was love at first sight. Roberts was transformed. He still didn't like to practice, but he was too afraid of Mr. Treadwell not to. There was something in his icy stare that generated fear in even the toughest band member, and more than a few were football players. He never physically ejected a student or harmed anyone for that matter, but everyone remembered that stare, that look, and that sick feeling inside when they were caught being any less than he demanded.

There was no life in Treadwell's stare now. He was totally dependent on those around him. His pressure and heart rate were supported by Roberts's drugs while his every breath came from the nurse handling the ambu bag. Once again the students were performing in concert for Mr. Treadwell.

Treadwell discovered and nourished hidden talent; but more important, he instilled self-confidence. It was in that band that Roberts learned that if he wanted something badly enough and worked hard enough, he could achieve it. In fact, in his senior year Treadwell asked him to try out for the all-state concert band. Roberts made it. He would never forget the smile on Treadwell's face. The band master had known all along that he could do it.

"Doctor Roberts, should we get the ventilator?" It was the nurse who was rhythmically squeezing the ambu bag that was restoring oxygen to Treadwell's brain.

"Yes," he answered simply, unable to take his eyes off the now dehumanized body before him. "Let's get him back to the critical care unit." He had acted instinctively up to this point, but now he felt the overwhelming desire to extricate himself from this nightmare. But he was in charge; he had to remain calm. "Thank you, everyone, it went just as we rehearsed it. I'd better talk to June."

He turned and walked slowly down the hall to the small family waiting room. Mrs. Treadwell sat in a darkened corner, arms encircling her chest. She was rocking back and forth in agony, but jumped expectantly to her feet as she heard him approach. Roberts moved to her quickly and put his arm around her shoulder.

"Is he . . . ?" She couldn't finish.

"Jim's had a serious heart attack. He's alive, but unconscious and in shock. We are breathing for him with a ventilator. I won't lie to you, it's not good."

"But he'll be okay?"

"I don't know, June. We've done all we can for him here. If there's anything more that can be done it will have to be in Iowa City. I think we should call them and have a helicopter flown up for him right away."

"Okay," she responded flatly. Her anxiety was turning to shock. "Can I see him?"

"Yes, I'll get one of the nurses to take you back. We're all so sorry. You know, most of us were his students." She didn't look up or respond and Roberts was relieved to get away. She was inconsolable and he hated this helpless feeling.

The next two hours were a blur. He called University Hospital and the helicopter was dispatched with one of the cardiology residents on board. Roberts divided the rest of his time between the patients in the office and his teacher in intensive care. The nurse called to report that Treadwell was seizing, so he returned to the unit. "Dammit," he sighed. "It looks like he may have had more brain damage than we thought. Let's get some IV Dilantin." Roberts added the Dilantin to the IV and stepped back, recalling concerts' finales and Mr. Treadwell's polite, self-assured bows to the applause.

By the time the helicopter could be heard overhead, Roberts was emotionally drained. Chances were remote that the town's band master would make it anywhere he was sent, and if he did, what would be left of his brilliant mind? Roberts wasn't able to stop the seizures.

Band Master

When the resident arrived, he looked at the twitching patient and let out his breath. "Jesus," he whispered and shook his head. Roberts felt he should apologize for not presenting a more stable candidate but remained silent wondering if somehow he could have done a better job. As his assistants readied Treadwell for transport, the resident mechanically performed his tasks. He studied the charts, checked the IV fluids, and took notes for the flight. Detached as he was, the cardiologist was now in charge. Roberts could do nothing but stand and watch, impotent. In life Treadwell had given him confidence, but in death had stolen a little of it away.

Roberts stood alone and continued to watch as the helicopter lifted off from the parking lot and headed north. The roar of the engine gradually became softer until, like the last note of a concert, it was barely heard . . . pianissimo. Roberts turned and walked back to the hospital with clenched fists shoved into his pockets, unable to hold back the tears streaming down his face.

SNAP JUDGMENTS

BY *Perri Klass, M.D.*

You work in an emergency room, one of the things you get good at is snap judgments. Walk into the room, size up the family. Rich, poor, with it, out of it. Caring, uncaring. People like them, people like us. That is to say, good parents and not so good parents. You know, competent, caring parents hovering anxiously over their sick little ones, distracting them with educational and safe toys in sturdy primary colors, singing them Raffi songs, versus the shiftless, heedless types, their own clothes smelling heavily of the cigarettes they've gone outside to smoke, the room smelling heavily of fast-food grease from the wrapping papers piled in the corner. The kind of people who don't bother to see their regular doctor before they come to the emergency room — maybe the kind of people who don't even *have* a regular doctor.

So it's two in the morning, and I hear the loving sound of the lullaby before I even enter the room. Two parents, one infant, and, boy, are they ever people-like-us. Well, like me. I mean, here I am with the long, frizzy hair and the bohemian earrings, the Cambridge, Massachusetts, academic earth mother as pediatrician, and here is this professorial bearded father and this ethnic-fabric-wrapped mother, and, sure enough, when I pick up the baby's chart, I can see that they too live in an academic town. No surprise.

Does it affect my manner? Well, it probably does; there's always a certain intensity when your patients remind you of yourself and your own family, at least for someone like me, who has always worked in hospitals and clinics where most of the patients weren't in that category. I look at these people and for an instant, in my somewhat-tired-but-not-yet-as-exhausted-as-I'm-gonna-be-by-morning mind, I feel recognition, bonding, and the little shiver that goes with every reminder that children are vulnerable, that into every family emergencies may fall. That is to say, as I recognize the cues of the mother's Indonesian earrings and the father's L. L. Bean backpack diaper bag leaning against the wall, I feel a quick flash of a reminder that there but for the grace of God. Could be me, could be my kid. A quick flash of gratitude that my kid is, in fact, safe at home, asleep, healthy. A renewed willingness to be right here, in this emergency room tonight, taking care of sick children — as long as my own can be safe at home, asleep, healthy. And so on. (That's the thing about the emergency room: snap judgments, snap emotions. Quick cues, quick responses. This all takes about a second and a half, but it all happens.)

I introduce myself, they look me over, I look at the baby. An all-cotton sleeper, naturally. Or rather, an all-cotton jumpsuit, probably contains a label saying specifically that it is not for use as sleepwear, since it won't have been treated with flame retardants. But then again, these are people who would never smoke, never allow anyone to smoke in their house, around their baby, and they are people who would rather let an infant sleep in 100 percent cotton than in any other fabric. I know all this, and guess how I know it.

The baby is little, but not newborn. Her name is Liane, and she's five months old, and she's awake and calm in her mother's arms. Doesn't look toxic. From here, from where I stand, doesn't look dehydrated, doesn't look in respiratory distress. Doesn't look like a disaster. But of course, something must have brought these people here in the middle of the night. Fever, vomiting, abdominal pain, first-time seizure? Seemed to be in terrible pain but now she's better? Maybe the classic, the croupy, barking cough that gets better as soon as you take the baby outside into the cold air?

And in fact, Liane's parents were talking about a cough. Never heard anything like it, her father said, shaking his head. It was so frightening, her mother said, and held the baby closer. A tear splashed down onto Liane's peaceful little face.

Croup, I thought, getting ready to give my croup talk. I would examine the baby, of course, listen to the history — but then I would end up giving them my croup talk. A viral infection, nothing we can do, antibiotics don't help, she'll fight it off herself. Turn on the humidifier, steam up the bathroom. Cold air helps. It'll be better in the morning.

I started to take the history. Well baby, born full-term. Had a sniffle now for a week or so, but eating well, no fever.

"Any trouble sleeping, does she wake up and cry like she's in pain?" I asked.

"Oh, no. She sleeps with us," her mother said, "and up till tonight she's been perfectly peaceful."

Well, naturally. Family bed. My own children eat white sugar and red meat, but I know the syndrome.

Then, tonight, this cough.

"You're not going to believe this cough," said the father.

"I was so scared," said the mother.

Meanwhile, I'd been in the room for ten minutes or so, and no cough. None at all.

Liane started to whimper, so her mother, of course, pulled up her shirt and clamped the baby onto the breast. A happy gurgle, a busily nursing baby. I would have to pry her off to examine her, of course, but the energy of her nursing told me plenty about the baby's general state of health.

Meanwhile, the father was busy over in the corner, digging in that backpack.

"So tell me about the cough," I said, thinking about the croup metaphors, the dog kennel, the seal pond.

Liane's father had taken a portable cassette tape recorder out of his backpack.

"I'll never be able to describe it," he said. "We decided to tape it so people would understand."

You did what? I thought, keeping on my face an expression of interest and encouragement: Taping your baby coughing, what a great idea! Wish we could get more people to do that!

He rewound the tape, then pressed PLAY. What came out of the tape recorder was his own voice, though, muffled, saying something about a meadow.

"He records his dreams," his wife said to me, matter-of-factly, while he fast-forwarded.

I nodded again. Sure he does. And a good thing, too.

And then he found the place: the cough. And, my God, what a cough it was. A tortured cascade of unstoppable hacking, the sound of a baby fighting desperately for breath against a paroxysm of remorseless coughing that sounded like it would turn the little body inside out. On and on it went, pouring out of the little tape player, while the baby herself nursed contentedly, on and on until it seemed to me, listening, that the baby on the tape must be dying, must be past what it could endure. And then, at the end — the whoop. I had read descriptions of the whoop, of course, but I had never heard a whoop, not a real one. And this was a real one. A strange high-pitched birdcall of a noise, a life-and-death noise of air rushing back in through a tightened airway. A noise so loud and terrifying that it brought two other doctors and a nurse to the door of the exam room to see what was happening.

So they looked in and saw the peaceful baby, and the tape

recorder kept turning, and once again we heard a sentence or two of the father's dreams.

"It's okay," I said, as he switched off the recorder. "Baby's fine."

After the others had dispersed, I turned back to the parents and said, trying hard to keep my question from sounding too accusatory, "Has Liane been immunized?"

Well, no, she hadn't. Not at all. They didn't believe in it. It wasn't natural, it wasn't safe.

I thought of a line of dialogue: Whooping cough may be natural, but it sure isn't safe. Didn't say it. In fact, the vaccine against whooping cough, or pertussis, is the most controversial of all the vaccines we give to children, controversial because it does provoke reactions in many children, and controversial because some researchers have blamed it for rare cases of neurologic damage and devastation. On the other hand, other studies have challenged even those rare bad outcomes, and the vaccine does prevent pertussis pretty well.

I changed the subject, unable to discuss this calmly. "Tell me what she looked like when she was coughing," I said, and they described the terrifying paroxysm, the little body contorted, the cough shaking her over and over and over.

"Did her lips change color?"

"Yes, at the end of one of those coughing spells, her lips looked all blue," her mother said, and began to cry in earnest. "I thought she was going to die."

So I admitted her to the hospital. Babies do die of pertussis, and a baby who turns blue at the end of a coughing paroxysm is a baby who needs oxygen and observation. It's true that her exam was pretty benign, true that we didn't really have much medicine to give her for her whooping cough, though we treated with erythromycin, which may shorten the symptoms — or at least the infectious period. The ward team was at first a little cynical about this vigorous healthy-appearing baby I wanted to admit. So I had her father play the tape again, volume turned up loud. This time the head of the ER came running, pushing a code cart. Pretty impressive.

The ward team admitted the baby, and the tape recorder, and went upstairs. Later on, I heard that every single pediatric resident in the hospital that night listened to the tape, and the next morning, some of the older attendings took the opportunity to pontificate a little about pertussis and the diseases of the past.

Except it wasn't a disease of the past. Not for Liane, who spent almost a week in the hospital, periodically coughing her guts out in her oxygen tent. It wasn't a disease of poverty and poor health care. It was a late-twentieth-century baby in the home of well-to-do, educated people, lying in her all-cotton sleeper in her smoke-free home, seized in the safety of her family bed by a wicked and dangerous and preventable illness. People like them, people like us.

CONTRIBUTORS

KEITH ABLOW is a psychiatrist in Chelsea, Massachusetts. His writing has appeared in the *Washington Post*. He has written several books, including *Without Mercy*, and is currently writing a novel for Pantheon Books.

ETHAN CANIN was a resident in Internal Medicine at the University of California Medical School at San Francisco. He is the bestselling author of *The Palace Thief*, *Emperor of the Air*, and *Blue River*.

TONY DAJER splits his time between his home in France and his job as an emergency physician in New York City. His writing appears regularly in *Discover* magazine. He is working on a book about Third World medicine.

DAVID FELDSHUH is Artistic Director at The Center for Theatre Arts at Cornell University. He trained in emergency medicine and works part-time as an emergency physician. Dr. Feldshuh's play, *Ms. Evers Boys*, was nominated for the Pulitzer Prize.

GLENN FLORES is Assistant Professor of Pediatrics and Public Health at Boston City Hospital. His writing has been featured in medical journals. He is currently working on a short story collection for publication as a book entitled *Hit the Road, Doc.*

PAMELA GRIM is an emergency physician at St. Vincent's Charity Hospital in Cleveland. Her writing has appeared in medical journals, as well as in the *North American Review*.

RICHARD HAIGHT is a family practitioner in Appleton, Wisconsin. His short stories have appeared in the magazines *M.D.* and *Hippocrates.*

ROD HAMER was a family practitioner and then an emergency physician. He is now semiretired and working in the student health center of the University of California at Santa Barbara.

TOM JANISSE is an anesthesiologist with Kaiser Permanente in Portland, Oregon. He has edited and published small-press literary magazines for fifteen years. His writing has been published in the *New England Journal of Medicine*.

MANJULA JEYAPALAN is a surgical resident at the University of California at Davis, in Oakland, California. She wrote *The Hunt* in medical school at the University of Iowa, for which she won a writing award from the Department of Medical Humanities.

PERRI KLASS is Assistant Professor of Pediatrics at Boston City Hospital and also works at the Dorchester House in Boston. Her short stories have been featured in multiple periodicals and *Best American Short Stories* anthologies. She has written several books, including *Baby Doctor*.

SIEGFRIED KRA is a cardiologist and Associate Clinical Professor at the Yale School of Medicine. He has written *The Three-Legged Stallion and Other Tales from a Doctor's Notebook* and medical texts for lay readers.

JOHN LANTOS is Associate Professor of Pediatrics and Medicine at the University of Chicago Pritzker School of Medicine and Associate Director of the Center for Clinical Medical Ethics at the University of Chicago. His writing has appeared in medical journals.

HAMISH MACLAREN is Clinical Head of the Emergency Department at Middlemore Hospital, in Auckland, New Zealand. His stories have been published in periodicals for general practitioners in New Zealand.

ROBERT MARION is Director of The Center for Congenital Disorders at Montefiore Medical Center in the Bronx and Associate Professor of Pediatrics at Albert Einstein College of Medicine. He has written three books, including *The Boy Who Felt No Pain* (winner of a 1991 Christopher Award).

STEWART MASSAD is Assistant Professor of Oncology in Obstetrics and Gynecology at Rush Presbyterian St. Luke's Medical Center in Chicago. He authored a book of short stories entitled *Doctors and Other Casualties*.

SUSAN MATES is a former concert violinist and an infectious disease specialist from Barrington, Rhode Island. Her collection of short stories, *The Good Doctor*, won the Iowa Short Fiction Award.

TOM MOSKALEWICZ is Medical Director of United Emergency Services, an emergency medical group in Wisconsin. His writing has been published in the *Wisconsin Medical Journal*.

JULIAN ORENSTEIN practices Emergency Medicine at Fairfax Hospital in Falls Church, Virginia.

MICHAEL PALMER is the bestselling author of medical thrillers, most recently *Critical Judgment*. He has practiced medicine for over twenty years, most recently as an emergency room physician. He is involved in the treatment of alcoholism and chemical dependence.

BARRY POLLACK is an emergency physician at Westlake Hospital in Westlake Village, California. He writes a column for Scripps Howard newspapers, served as medical adviser to the hit medical series *St. Elsewhere*, and wrote episodes of *Trapper John, M.D.*

MICKEY ZUCKER REICHERT is a pediatrician at Community Health Care in Davenport, Iowa. She has written numerous science fiction and fantasy books, and recently *The Unknown Soldier*.

LAWRENCE SCHNEIDERMAN is a professor in the Department of Family and Preventive Medicine at The University of California at San Diego. His short stories and plays have appeared widely. He won the Dramalogue Award, and authored *Sea Nymphs by the Hour*.

RICHARD SELZER retired from his position as Professor of Surgery at Yale Medical School to devote himself full time to writing. He is the author of numerous books of essays and short stories, most recently *Raising the Dead*.

SAMUEL SHEM is the pen name of a Boston-area psychiatrist, novelist, and playwright. In addition to several plays, he wrote *The House of God*, a novel about medical internship that has sold more than one million copies.

JOHN STONE founded the Emergency Medicine Residency Program at Emory University School of Medicine. He is a cardiologist as well as Associate Dean and Director of Admissions at the medical school. He has authored three volumes of poetry, most recently *In the Country of Hearts.*

JAMES THOMAS practices Emergency Medicine at Cottage Hospital in Santa Barbara, California.

DAN SACHS is an emergency physician in Chicago. He completed the residency program in Emergency Medicine at Christ Hospital & Medical Center, a level-1 trauma center in Cook County, Chicago.

Acknowledgments

Acknowledgments

254